SAUNDERS

HEALTH

PROFESSIONAL'S

Planner

SAUNDERS

An Imprint of Elsevier

SAUNDERS
An Imprint of Elsevier
The Curtis Center
Independence Square West
Philadelphia, Pennsylvania 19106-3399

Saunders Health Professional's Planner   ISBN 0-7216-9571-X

Printed in the United States of America

Last digit is the print number: 9 8 7 6 5 4 3 2

NOTICE

Allied Health is an ever-changing field. Standard safety precautions must be followed but as new research and clinical experience broaden our knowledge, changes in treatment and drug therapy become necessary or appropriate. Readers are advised to check the product information currently provided by the manufacturer of each drug to be administered to verify the recommended dose, the methods and duration of administration and the contraindications. It is the responsibility of the treating physician, relying on experience and knowledge of the patient, to determine dosages and the best treatment for the patient. Neither the publisher nor the editor assumes any responsibility for any injury and/or damage to persons or property.

Publisher's Foreword

In speaking with students, allied health program directors, instructors and clinical coordinators, we found that people were looking for a planner and guide that would assist in organizing time and information for students in health professions. With the Saunders Health Professional's Planner, students can:

➤ Keep track of activities, assignments and goals.
➤ Apply material learned in career development and study skills texts
➤ Build a dynamic resume with less stress
➤ Carry key information helpful to a variety of health professions
➤ Carry calendar and "To Do" information along with useful resource information

The Saunders Health Professional's Planner has six sections:

1. Quick Review/Orientation
2. Quick Reference
3. Planner—Wide Angle View (including Monthly Planner)
4. Planner—Detailed View (Weekly Planner)
5. Directory/Address Book
6. Career Planner (including resume building and interview forms)

Additional Key Features:

➤ **Useful Reference Material geared specifically toward Health Professions**

Includes key information in tables and lists for easy reference. This makes it simple to find important information since it is combined with the planner.

➤ **Quick Math Review**

Brief math review reference, describing and demonstrating many of the most common math operations. Imagine having math anxiety diminished in a calendar/planner you can carry in a lab coat!

➢ **Resume Builder Forms and Job Search Tools**

The series of Resume Builder Forms allows you to keep a running tab of special accomplishments, key experiences, and job duties. You can add to these forms throughout your courses and then use these forms to easily create a dynamic resume. And there are even forms to help you do your best in an interview!

➢ **Useful Tracking Forms**

Use the forms in the Saunders Health Professional's Planner to set and accomplish your goals, track your performance, and organize your assignments!

Saunders Health Professional's Planner Table of Contents

Section 3   Planner—Wide Angle View

Section 4   Planner—Detailed View

Section 5   Career Planner

Section 6   Directory/Address Book

Math Review

Basic Operations

Operation	What to Do	Examples
Fractions		
Reducing fractions	Find a number that divides evenly into both the numerator and the denominator. You may have to do this more than once if you want it to be at its lowest terms (meaning that there are no other numbers by which both can be evenly divided).	18/30 Both 18 and 30 can be divided evenly by 2, resulting in 9/15 Both 9 and 15 can be divided evenly by 3, resulting in 3/5 (This can also be done in one step by dividing 18 and 30 by 6 = 3/5.)
Changing fractions so that they share the lowest common denominator	1. Find the smallest number that can be evenly divided by all the denominators in a series of fractions. This is the new denominator. 2. Divide the new denominator by the original denominator. 3. Multiply the product from step 2 times the numerator. This number is the new numerator.	By trial and error, we discover that the lowest common denominator for 1/6, 3/4, and 5/8 is 24. To convert 1/6, divide 24 by 6. The answer is 4. Multiply 4 times the numerator, 1. The new fraction is 4/24. To convert 3/4: 24 divided by 4 = 6 6 × 3 = 18 New fraction is 18/24 To convert 5/8: 24 divided by 8 = 3 3 × 5 = 15 New fraction is 15/24
Simplifying improper fractions	Divide the numerator by the denominator. If there is a remainder (R), it is the numerator of the fraction. The denominator is the same as in the improper fraction. Reduce the fraction, if necessary.	10/4 is improper because the numerator is larger than the denominator. 10 divided by 4 = 2 R 2 2 2/4 = 2 1/2

Continued

Basic Operations *(continued)*

Operation	What to Do	Examples
	Fractions (continued)	
Adding and subtracting	1. If the fractions do not have the same denominator, find the lowest common denominator. 2. Add or subtract the numerators. 3. Use the common denominator in the answer. 4. Simplify the result if it is an improper fraction. Caution: When subtracting mixed numbers, it is best to change them to improper fractions before subtracting the numerators.	1/6 + 3/4 + 5/8 = ? 24 is the lowest common denominator. 4/24 + 18/24 + 15/24 = 37/24. 37/24 is an improper fraction, so divide 37 by 24 by 1 R 13. 37/24 = 1 13/24 5/8 − 1/4 = ? 8 is the lowest common denominator. 5/8 − 2/8 = 3/8
Multiplying fractions	1. Multiply the numerators and then the denominators. 2. Reduce the fraction, if necessary.	1/2 × 3/4 = ? 1 × 3 = 3 2 × 4 = 8
Dividing fractions (everyone's big fear!)	1. Invert (switch) the numerator and the denominator of the divisor. 2. Multiply the numerators and the denominators. (That's right—you don't actually divide as we know it. This is what makes an otherwise simple operation seem confusing and hard to remember.) 3. If necessary, simplify to a proper fraction.	3/4 divided by 1/2 = ? Invert: 1/2 becomes 2/1 3 × 2 = 6 4 × 1 = 4 6/4 is an improper fraction. 6 divided by 4 = 1 R 2 = 1 2/4 = 1 1/2

Continued

Basic Operations *(continued)*

Operation	What to Do	Examples
Decimals		
Adding and subtracting decimals	1. Line up the numbers so that the decimal points are aligned. 2. Use zeros to fill in the spaces to the right of the decimal point. 3. Add or subtract as you would any numbers. 4. Place the decimal point in the answer directly under the points in the numbers you added or subtracted.	To add 3.96, 4.229 and 6.1: 3.960 4.229 6.100 14.289 To subtract 18.453 from 72.5: 72.500 − 18.453 54.047
Multiplying decimals	1. Multiply as you would whole numbers. 2. Count and total the digits to the right of the decimal point in each factor. 3. Place the decimal point in the answer that total number of spaces from the right. 4. Insert zeros as needed for placement of the decimal point.	16.953 × 3.502 59.369406
Dividing decimals	1. Set up the problem like any division problem. 2. If the divisor is a decimal, move the decimal point to the right and place it immediately following the last digit in the number. Then move the decimal point in the dividend to the right the same number of spaces. Add zeros if necessary. 3. Divide the numbers. 4. Place the decimal point in the answer directly above the decimal point in the dividend.	2.5/10 2.5⌐10.0 4.0 25⌐100.0

Continued

4 *Quick Review Section*

Math Review

Basic Operations *(continued)*

Operation	What to Do	Examples
Decimals and Fractions		
Changing decimals to fractions	1. Write the numbers in the decimal as the numerator. 2. Write the unit of the decimal as the denominator (tenths, hundredths, thousandths, etc). 3. Reduce the fraction, if necessary.	$0.25 = ?$ Numerator is 25 0.25 has two places; therefore, use 100 for the denominator. $0.25 = 25/100$ Both 25 and 100 can be evenly divided by 25: $\dfrac{25 \div 25}{100 \div 25} = \dfrac{1}{4}$ $0.25 = 1/4$
Changing fractions to decimals	1. Set up a division problem in which the numerator is divided by the denominator. 2. Before dividing, check to see if the numerator is smaller than the denominator. If it is, write a decimal point and one or more zeros, as needed.	$2/3 = ?$ 3 2 $3\overline{)2.00}$ add decimal point and zeros $\begin{array}{r}.66\\3\overline{)2.00}\\\underline{18\times}\\20\end{array}$
Percentages		
Changing percentages to decimals	1. Start counting from the decimal point and move it 2 places to the left. Fill in with zeros as needed. (Note: If the whole number does not have a decimal point written in, it is understood to be located at the far right side of the number.) 2. Drop the percent sign.	To change 41% to a decimal: The decimal point is understood to be to the right of the 1 $41\% = 41.0\%$ Move the decimal point 2 places to the left: 0.41 $41\% = 0.41$ To change 3% to a decimal: The decimal point is understood to be to the right of the 3. $3\% = 3.0\%$ Move the decimal point 2 places to the left: 0.03 $3\% = 0.03$

Continued

Basic Operations *(continued)*

Operation	What to Do	Examples
Percentages (continued)		
Calculating amounts represented by percentages	1. Change the percent to a decimal. 2. Multiply the whole number by the decimal. 3. Count and total the digits to the right of the decimal point in the multiplier. 4. Place the decimal point in the answer that total number of spaces from the right. (Extra zeros on the far right may be dropped.)	To find 65% of 730: $65\% = 0.65$ $\begin{array}{r} 730 \\ \times\ 0.65 \\ \hline 474.50 \end{array}$ 65% of 730 = 474.5
Equations		
Solving simple equations	1. Your goal is to find the value of an unknown quantity (x). You do this by reorganizing the equation so the unknown is by itself on one side of the equals sign. 2. Isolate x by adding, subtracting, multiplying, or dividing both sides of the equation in the same way. (You must always treat both sides of an equation the same way.) 3. You may have to do more than one calculation to isolate x completely. Note: Positive and negative numbers cancel each other out.	$5 + x = 12$ You want x by itself, so you need to eliminate the 5. Subtract 5 from both sides of the equation. $5 + x -\ 5 = 12 -\ 5$ $x = 7$ $6x -\ 3 = 15$ Add 3 to each side: $6x -\ 3 +\ = 15 + 3$ $6x = 18$ Divide each side by 6: $6x/6 = 18/6$ $x = 3$

Continued

Basic Operations *(continued)*

Operation	What to Do	Examples
	Proportions	
Finding an unknown quantity in a proportion	1. Substitute x for the unknown quantity.	1:2 = 10:x
		1/2= 10/x
	2. Write each of the 2 ratios as fractions.	1 × x = 2 × 10
		x = 20
	3. Multiply the denominators by the opposite numerators.	Therefore, 1:2 = 10:20
		8:x = 14:91
	4. Solve for x.	8/x = 14/91
	5. Write out the completed proportion.	8 × 91 = 14 × x
		728 = 14x
		728/14 = 14x/14
	Note: Another common way to discuss proportions is in terms of the "means" and the "extremes." In the example 1:2 = 10:x, 1 and x are the extremes and 2 and 10 are the means.	x = 52
		Therefore, 8:52 = 14:91
		1:2 = 10:x
		mean
		extreme
		Multiply the means and extremes:
		1 × x = 2 × 10
		x = 20
	The product of the means equals the product of the extremes. This is the same operation as cross-multiplying the fractions.	Therefore, 1:2 = 10:20
		8:x = 14:91
		Multiply the means and extremes:
		8 × 91 = x × 14
		14x = 728
		Isolate x:
		14x/14 = 728/14
		x = 52
		Therefore, 8:52 = 14:91

From: Haroun, L. (2000), *Career Development for Health Professionals.* Phila. : W B Saunders, p. 140-143. Reprinted with permission.

Multiplication Chart

	1	2	3	4	5	6	7	8	9	10	11	12
1	1	2	3	4	5	6	7	8	9	10	11	12
2	2	4	6	8	10	12	14	16	18	20	22	24
3	3	6	9	12	15	18	21	24	27	30	33	36
4	4	8	12	16	20	24	28	32	36	40	44	48
5	5	10	15	20	25	30	35	40	45	50	55	60
6	6	12	18	24	30	36	42	48	54	60	66	72
7	7	14	21	28	35	42	49	56	63	70	77	84
8	8	16	24	32	40	48	56	64	72	80	88	96
9	9	18	27	36	45	54	63	72	81	90	99	108
10	10	20	30	40	50	60	70	80	90	100	110	120
11	11	22	33	44	55	66	77	88	99	110	121	132
12	12	24	36	48	60	72	84	96	108	120	132	144

Knowing the products of all possible combinations of the numbers 1 through 12 is a great time saver. This is not a substitute for learning how to multiply but a way to increase your efficiency. It is also a good study aid for learning the multiplication tables. To use the chart, find the intersection of the two numbers you wish to multiply, one from the row across the top and the other from the far left column. For example, to multiply 3 times 4, find the 3 in the top row and the 4 in the first column. Move down from the 3 and across from the 4 until the lines meet at 12. This is the answer. Study from the table or make flashcards for any combinations you need to memorize. You can also use graph paper to set up blank tables to fill in to review and quiz yourself.

The multiplication table can also be used as a tool to reduce fractions if the numerator and denominator appear in the same column. For example, for 12/96, follow both 12 and 96 to the far left column: 12 becomes 1 and 96 becomes 8; 12/96 = 1/8. The fraction may need to be reduced further. For example, 24/48 = 2/4; 2/4 can be further reduced to 1/2.

From: Haroun, L. (2000). Career Development for Health Professionals Phila.: W B Saunders, p. 144. Reprinted with permission.

The Language of Math

Word or Phrase	What it Means	Examples
Digit	Any of the numerals 0 to 9.	The number 8 3 4 has three digits: 8, 3, and 4.
Factors	The numbers being multiplied in a multiplication problem.	8 × 10 = 80 8 and 10 are the factors
Product	The answer to a multiplication problem.	8 × 10 = 80 80 is the product
Fraction	Used to represent equal parts of a whole. Always written as two numbers, one on top of the other.	1/2 represents 1 of the 2 equal parts into which a whole of something has been divided. 5/12 represents 5 of the 12 equal parts into which a whole has been divided.
Numerator	The top number in a fraction. It tells you how many pieces of the whole you have.	In the fraction 1/2, 1 is the numerator. In 5/12, 5 is the numerator.
Denominator	The bottom number in a fraction. It tells you into how many equal pieces a whole has been divided. The larger the number, the smaller the pieces.	In 1/2, 2 is the denominator. In 5/12, 12 is the denominator.
Proper Fraction	A fraction in which the numerator is smaller than the denominator.	3/4 3 is smaller than 4
Improper Fraction	A fraction in which the numerator is larger than the denominator.	4/3 4 is larger than 3. This represents a whole number and a fraction: 1 1/3. (There are 3 thirds in a whole, which equals 1. 1/3 represents the additional—or 4th—third.)

Continued

The Language of Math *(continued)*

Word or Phrase	What it Means	Examples
Lowest Common Denominator	The smallest number that can be evenly divided (no remainder) by all the denominators in a series of fractions. It is necessary to find this number when you want to add or subtract fractions.	The lowest common denominator for 1/6, 3/4, and 5/8 is 24. 24 divided by 6 = 4 24 divided by 4 = 6 24 divided by 8 = 3
Simplest Form	A fraction in which the numerator and denominator cannot be evenly divided by the same number.	1/2 is the simplest form for the following fractions: 2/4, 3/6, 4/8, 5/10, 25/50
Decimal	Special fractions. They are written with decimal points, the same symbol as a period. When decimals are written as fractions, they always have denominators written in units of 10 (10, 100, 1000, 10,000, etc.).	0.3 = 3/10. Both represent 3 of the 10 equal parts of a whole.
Whole Number	A number that has no fraction or decimal.	5, 67, and 1893 are whole numbers.
Mixed Number	A number that has two parts: a whole number and a fraction.	1 1/3, 4 1/2, 17 2/5
Percentage	A fraction with a denominator of 100 which is expressed as a whole number with a percent sign.	37% represents 37 of the 100 parts of a whole. It is the same as 37/100 and 0.37.
Cubic Measurement	Measure of volume, or the amount of space that something takes up. Medications are sometimes measured in cubic centimeters.	To calculate the volume of a box, multiply the height times the width times the length. A box that is 3 feet long, 2 feet high, and 5 feet wide = 3 × 2 × 5 = 30 cubic feet.

Continued

The Language of Math *(continued)*

Word or Phrase	What it Means	Examples
Dividend	In a division problem, the number to be divided.	8)64 ← dividend
Divisor	The number by which the dividend is divided in a division problem.	8)64 divisor
Ratio	Expresses the relationship of 2 numbers. They can be written several ways.	The relationship between 1 and 2 can be written as 1 to 2, 1:2, or 1/2.
Proportion	Statement that 2 ratios are equal.	1:2 = 5:10 1/2 = 5/10 (1 is to 2 as 5 is to 10)
Equation	Statement which says that 2 quantities are equal. This equality is represented by an "equals" sign. Equations are used to help you find values for unknown quantities by using the information you do know. The unknown quantities are commonly represented by letters.	$x + 12 = 18$ $6x - 4 = 30 + 26$
Place Value Chart	A chart that shows the unit values of the places that follow the decimal point.	Tenths: 0.1 Hundredths: 0.01 Thousandths: 0.001 Ten thousandths: 0.0001 Hundred thousandths: 0.00001

From: Haroun, L. (2000). Career Development for Health Professionals Phila.: W B Saunders, p.138-139, Table 6-1. Reprinted with permission.

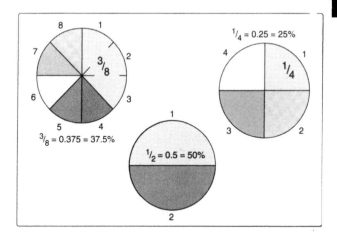

Relationship of fractions, decimals, and percentages.

How the Metric System Works

Type of Measurement	Units of Measurement	How it Compares With the US System
Length or Distance	*meter* (m) = basic unit	A little more than 1 yard (1 yard = 36 inches and 1 meter = 39.37 inches)
	millimeter (mm) = 0.001 meter	About the size of the width of a pinhead. There are just over 25 millimeters in 1 inch.
	centimeter (cm) = 0.01 meter	About 2/5 (or 0.4) of an inch, the width of a child's little finger. There are about 2 1/2 centimeters in an inch.
	decimeter (dm) = 0.1 meter	About 4 inches
	dekameter (dam) = 10 meters	A little more than 10 yards
	hectometer (hm) = 100 meters	A little more than 100 yards
	kilometer (km) = 1000 meters	About 3/5 (or 0.62) of a mile
Liquids or Volume	*liter* (L) = basic unit	Approximately 1 quart (2 liters is now a popular-sized soft drink bottle; that's about 1/2 gallon because there are 4 quarts in a gallon)
	*milliliter** (mL) = 0.001 liter	*Very* small drop (commonly used in medicine)
	centiliter (cL) = 0.01 liter	About 2 teaspoons
	deciliter (dL) = 0.1 liter	Between 1/3 and 1/2 cup
	dekaliter (daL) = 10 liters	About 10 quarts or 2 1/2 gallons
	hectoliter (hL) = 100 liters	About 25 gallons
	kiloliter (kL) = 1000 liters	About 250 gallons

Continued

How the Metric System Works *(continued)*

Type of Measurement	*Units of Measurement*	*How it Compares With the US System*
Weight or Mass of Solids	*gram* (Gm, g) = basic unit	Approximately 1/28 of an ounce. About the weight of a paperclip.
	microgram (mcg) = 0.000001 gram	An incredibly small amount (1 millionth of 1/400 of a pound!) Don't be fooled, however. This can be a significant amount in health care. The body depends on very small quantities of certain substances to function properly. It can also be harmed by minute amounts of the wrong substances.
	milligram (mg) = 0.001 gram	Also very small amounts, although they are many times heavier than a microgram.
	centigram (cg) = 0.01 gram	
	decigram (dg) = 0.1 gram	
	dekagram (dag) = 10 grams	5/14 of an ounce
	hectogram (hg) = 100 grams	About 3 1/2 ounces
	kilogram (kg) = 1000 grams	2.2 pounds

Continued

How the Metric System Works *(continued)*

Type of Measurement	Units of Measurement	How it Compares With the US System
Temperature	Celsius (commonly called centigrade) 0° C = freezing point of water 100° C = boiling point of water	Fahrenheit is the system commonly used in the United States. In this system, 32° F is freezing and 95° F is a sunny day at the beach.
	Celsius thermometers are marked in one-tenth intervals.	1° C = 1.8 times 1° F
	Water freezes: 0° C	32° F
	Normal body temperature: 37° C	98.6° F
	Water boils: 100° C	212° F
	Sterilization occurs: 121° C	250° F
	To convert between the 2 systems:	
	Fahrenheit to Celsius: 1. Subtract 32 from the F temperature 2. Multiply by 5/9	98.6° F 98.6 − 32 = 66.6 5/9 × 66.6 = 5/9 × 66.6/1.0 = 37
	Celsius to Fahrenheit: 1. Multiply the C temperature by 9/5 2. Add 32	37 × 9/5 = 37/1 × 9/5 = 333/5 = 66.6 66.6 + 32 = 98.6

*A milliliter is the same amount as a cubic centimeter (cc). This is important to know in health care because these terms are sometimes used interchangeably.

From: Haroun, L. (2000). Career Development for Health Professionals Phila.: W B Saunders, p. 146-147, Table 6-3. Reprinted with permission.

Taking Notes & Studying

Notes on Taking Great Notes

Listen for organizational patterns. There are some common ways that health care topics are presented, and recognizing these can help you follow your instructor more easily and improve your note taking.

A. Clusters of information: topics are divided into chunks of related material. A lecture covers one chunk before moving on to the next. Examples: the human body parts and functions are usually grouped by systems: skeletal, digestive, and reproductive. Appointment scheduling for the medical office is usually organized by the different methods used to set them.

B. Procedures: these are often explained in a step-by-step sequence. Examples include how to measure an infant and how to perform one-person, adult CPR.

C. Concepts or procedures with rationale: material is introduced, and then important reasons are given to explain and support it. Examples: legal reasons for maintaining patient confidentiality; why standard precautions must be followed.

D. Definitions: in addition to medical terminology, each area of health care has its own vocabulary. Lectures may be organized around explanations of new terms. Example: discussion of terms related to medical insurance billing.

E. How things work: descriptions and explanations. Examples: parts and operation of the microscope; safe use of the autoclave.

F. Lists: descriptions or explanations of a number of items of equal importance. Examples: purpose and interpretation of a series of lab tests; different medications and their use.

Continued

G. Patterns created by the instructor: material presented in a specific order. Example: anatomy and physiology course in which body systems are always presented in the same order—names of parts; purpose and function of each part; common disorders; causes; diagnostic tests; treatments; prevention.

H. Verbal signals: certain words tell you where the lecture is going. Examples: "Let's go on to . . ." signals the transition to a new topic. "Therefore" and "In conclusion" let you know that a summary statement is coming. "First," "second," and so on advise you that there will be a list of items of equal importance.

From: Haroun, L. (2000). Career Development for Health Professionals Phila.: W B Saunders, p.77, Roman III (A-H). Reprinted with permission.

More Ideas for Taking Great Notes

1. Be there! Do your best to be present for both the beginning and end of lectures. Introductions and conclusions often contain valuable information about what the instructor considers to be most important. Conclusions may clarify points that seemed fuzzy or unrelated earlier in the lecture.

2. Leave some blank space between the major ideas or clusters of related information so that you can make additions when you edit and review. You may think of something you forgot to write down or find helpful explanations in your textbook or other sources. If you have trouble understanding the material or if you get lost and have gaps in your notes, leave a lot of space to fill in later.

3. Write out examples, definitions, formulas, and calculations.

4. Write on only one side of the paper so that you can lay the pages out to relate information and review. Some students use blank facing pages to create study notes.

5. Do your best to write down words you do not know. Guess at the spelling and circle the words so that you can look up their meanings or ask the instructor.

Taking Notes

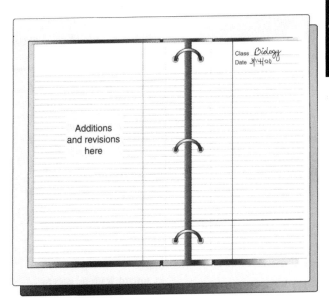

Use the facing page or reverse side of your note pages to write additions or revisions.

From: Haroun, L. (2000). Career Development for Health Professionals Phila.: W B Saunders, p. 83, incl. 4-3, cont. onto p. 84. Reprinted with permission.

6. Write as neatly as possible. Practice improving your handwriting if necessary. Try printing if it does not slow you down too much. Aim for a balance between speed and legibility. Recopying notes to make them neater takes time that you could use more productively. There are, however, a few circumstances in which rewriting typing, ar word processing notes is recommended. If you have strong keyboarding skills, you may find that this process serves as a good review of the lecture. If you are a kinesthetic learner, you may benefit from the activity of keyboarding. Finally, on those few occasions when your notes are a total disaster, it may be worth your time to clean them up. Keep in mind that good handwriting is important on the job because the quality of patient care depends on the ability of other health professionals to read your written documentation. Because

Continued

many records are summoned to court, their legibility can be critical in defending the actions of health care personnel.

7. Erasable pens are good for note taking, although regular pens can be used if you make corrections neatly. Pencils can break or need sharpening, and the writing tends to fade and smudge over time.

8. Create a set of symbols to mark your notes as you take them. Here are some ideas:

   T = test item (instructor announced or hinted).

   ?? = got lost and need to fill in later.

   P = personal thoughts: your own ideas that you want to jot down before you forget. (Or you can bracket your own thoughts to distinguish them from what the instructor says.)

   J = important for job success, something employers look for.

9. Develop abbreviations to increase your recording speed. Use standard abbreviations or invent your own—or use a combination. See table for suggestions.

From: Haroun, L. (2000). Career Development for Health Professionals Phila.: W B Saunders, p. 83, incl. 4-3, cont. onto p. 84 Reprinted with permission.

Developing Abbreviations for Note Taking: Standard Abbreviations

Word	Standard Abbreviation
and	&
and so forth	etc
equals, same as, means	=
for example	eg
less than	<
more than	>
negative	−
not the same as, does not equal	≠
number	#
of, per	/
positive	+
regarding	re
therefore	∴
times	×
to, toward, leads to, goes to	→
versus	vs
with	w/ or $\bar{c}$
without	w/o or $\bar{s}$

Spell words as they sound, leaving out silent letters

Examples	Phonetic Spelling
	(Finally, spelling just like its sound!)
although	altho
through	thru

Shorten words by leaving out the vowels

Word	Shortened Form
blood	bld
book	bk
homework	hmwrk
learn	lrn
patient	pt

Continued

Develop your own short forms of common words

Word	Shortened Form
anatomy	anat
appointment	appt
because	bec
determine	det
important	imp
information	info
introduction	intro
necessary	nec
procedure	proc
psychology	psych
venipuncture	venip

Learn common medical abbreviations

Word	Abbreviation
cardiopulmonary resuscitation	CPR
electrocardiography	EKG
medical assistant	MA
occupational therapy	OT

From: Haroun, L. (2000). Career Development for Health Professionals. Phila.: W B Saunders, p. 84-85 Table 4-1. Reprinted with permission.

A Guidesheet for Literature Searching

Analyze your topic using this guidesheet, checking all aspects of it that you may want to address. Examine quickly each of the suggested sources, to determine if you should use it. Decide which tools may be most productive. Work carefully with each of these tools.

By Topic

Business	*Hospital Literature Index*, CD + Health
Drugs	*Index Medicus*, CD + MEDLINE
	International Pharmaceutical Abstracts
	MICROMEDEX
Education	ERIC (CD)
	Consumer Health & Nutrition Index
	Specialty index—professionals
	PsychologicalAbstracts, PsycLIT (CD)
Ethics	*Bibliography of Bioethics*

History	*Bibliography of the History of Medicine* (remember history subheading in MeSH)
Law	*Hospital Literature Index,* CD + Health *Bibliography of Bioethics*
Management/ Administration	*Abstracts of Health Care Management Studies*
Pathophysiology	*Index Medicus,* CD + MEDLINE *Science Citation Index* *Current Contents: Clinical Medicine*
Popular topics	*Reader's Guide to Periodical Literature* *Consumer Health & Nutrition Index*
Psychology	*PsychologicalAbstracts,* PsycLIT (CD) *Social Science Citation Index* *Current Contents: Social & Behavioral Sciences*
Religion	*PsychologicalAbstracts,* PsycLIT (CD) *Social Science Citation Index*
Technology	*Index Medicus,* CD + MEDLINE

By Time
Associations
Current contents
Institutions
Newspapers
Personal contacts
Other print tools

By Type of Material

Books	Books in Print *Medical and Health Care Books and Serials in Print*
Definitions	Dictionaries Encyclopedias
Journal articles	miniMEDLINE CD-ROM databases Various indexes and abstracts
Numbers/ Statistics	miniMEDLINE *American Statistics Index*
Pamphlets	Telephone book "Blue Pages" Pamphlet File
People/Contacts	*Encyclopedia of Associations*

From: Miller/Keane: Encyclopedia & Dictionary of Medicine, Nursing, & Allied Health (6th ed.). Philadelphia: WB Saunders, p. 1913. Reprinted with permission.

Charting

Documentation (Charting) Guidelines

Think of your charting as a camera that takes the patient's picture.

Organize Your Thoughts

- What have I seen that relates to this problem?
- What have I done about it?
- What do I plan to do about it?
- How has my patient responded to what has been done?

Build Your Planning On

- Your initial assessment and further findings.
- Your indentification of the patient's problems.
- Your patient care.

General Guidelines

1. Chart neatly, legibly, and in blue or black ink.
2. Be brief, concise, accurate, and complete.
3. Use good grammar, correct spelling, correct punctuation, and proper terminology.
4. Note the time of each entry; also include month, date, year at the beginning of the shift charting.
5. Use a new line for each "new" (timed) entry. Put an ink line through extra space on the line you are charting on if you haven't used the entire line.
6. DO NOT ERASE. Draw a single line through an error, write "incorrect," "error," or "mistaken" entry over it and sign your initials (check agency procedure).
7. Never chart in advance of doing something; particularly do not chart medications before they are administered.
8. Include your signature and student designation (i.e., "S.N."). Use first initial and last name with that designation.

Continued

9. Leave out the word *Patient*. If the meaning of the entry is ambiguous, use the patient's name.
10. Use only those abbreviations accepted in your hospital (see the documentation manual).
11. Retain recopied pages in the back of the chart (i.e., corrected graphic record).
12. Check on correct format for charting in your clinical facility.
13. Use flow sheets whenever possible—don't duplicate the information in the nurse's notes.
14. Use easily defined terms (e.g., "ate 75%, of meal," rather than "ate well").
15. Rather than "tolerated well," state outcome: tolerated without pain, without nausea, or without complaint. ("Well" means different things to each of us.)

Content to Include

Body Care: Type of bath, back care, skin care and assessment, mouth care, hair care, perineal care, position changes (most data goes on flow sheets)

Intake: Diet, amount eaten, fluids (oral, NG, IV); IV site condition, type of fluid, equipment changed, complaints (use activity sheet, I & O sheet, IV flow sheet)

Output: Emesis, B.M., wound drainage, urine, vaginal flow, perspiration; include amounts and appearance (I & O sheet, nurse's notes)

Treatments: Time, type, duration, appearance of area treated, special equipment, specifics of procedures: how it is done, patient response. If left unit, time left, and by which conveyance; time returned

Tests: Laboratory specimens drawn; cultures, disposition of specimens, X-rays, sonograms, endoscopies, patient reaction, outcome if known, time left and returned to floor

Dressings: Appearance of incision or wound, smell, presence of drainage and appearance, how redressed and by whom

Activity: Time, ambulation and distance, exercises performed, including leg and breathing postoperatively, range of motion (ROM) performed, physical therapy, condition of pressure points, repositioning and for how long, and patient response to each

Oxygen: Time applied or amount changed, method of administration, safety precautions

Medications: Time, amount, route, response, any adverse reaction or side effects, omission or delay, evidence of expected action (PRN and STAT doses are charted on the medication administration record [MAR] as well as the nurse's notes)

Sleep: Day or night; amount, interruptions; patient comments

Mental State: Mood, level of consciousness, general behavior (be objective)

Preoperative Preparation: Teaching, physical preparation, time and by whom; patient questions

Special Conditions: Traction, cast, special equipment— time applied, condition of patient, circulation checks and findings, skin condition, smell

Vital Signs: Temperature, pulse, respiration, blood pressure; weight (on graphic record)

Doctor's Visits: Examinations and treatments

Visitors: Who, how long, patient reaction

Feelings: What patient states regarding feelings, complaints, concerns

Physical Assessment: What you see, hear, smell, and feel: Auscultation of lungs, heart, bowel sounds, palpation of abdomen and pulses; inspection of skin, assessment of problem area in depth

Safety Factors: Side rails up or down, replaced after working with patient; warnings; restraints in place

From: DeWit, S.(1999). Saunders Student Nurse Planner (Version 2). Philadelphia: WB Saunders, p.52-52 Table 2-9. Reprinted with Permission.

Quick Chart Review

Sheet	Information
Face Sheet	Marital status, age, insurance coverage, occupation, significant others, religion, location of home
Physician's Order Sheet (admitting day up to today)	Tests ordered, medications, intravenous solutions, treatments to be done
Physician's History and Physical	Overview of total health status and summary of current health problems; allergies
Physician's Progress Notes	Gives clues to future tests and orders; status of problems
Nursing Admission Assessment	Medications taken at home, allergies; prosthetic devices such as hearing aid, glasses; previous health problems and hospitalizations, previous surgeries, and so forth
Laboratory Reports	Tests that have been completed, results, and normal values
Other Test Results	Findings that are abnormal (read the conclusions); pathology reports tell whether patient has cancer
Medication Sheets	Medications ordered; how often patient is taking PRN medications and what they are
Consultation Sheets	Conclusions of other members of the health care team
Nurse's Notes	Care given for previous 24 hours; problems encountered; changes in plan of care; visitors, psychological outlook
Flow Sheets	Vital signs, intake and output, intravenous fluids, blood administered, neurologic signs and changes, and so forth
Nursing Care Plan, Care Pathway, or "Needs" List	Lists the problems or nursing diagnoses, with goals and interventions to be done
Operative Report	Conclusion tells what was done; abnormalities found and problems encountered

From: DeWit, S.(1999). Saunders Student Nurse Planner (Version 2). Philadelphia: WB Saunders, p. 24, Table 2-1. Reprinted with Permission.

Goals

Goals—Your Signposts to Success

Goals are based on your mission statement and provide
guidance for your journey through life. Values provide the
"why" for your actions, your mission statement the "what,"
and goals the "how." Goals serve as signposts, giving your
life direction and measuring your progress on the road to
success. Use them to motivate yourself and mark your
accomplishments.

The Marks of a Good Goal

Good goals share the following characteristics:

- In line with your values: Do they agree with your
  basic beliefs?

- Reasonable: Do you have adequate time, energy, and
  knowledge?

- Measurable: How will you know if you have achieved
  them?

- Clearly stated: Will you understand your intention
  next month?

- Written: Have you thought them out and committed
  them to paper?

- Worth your time: Will they help you fulfill your
  mission?

Here are two examples of well-stated goals for a health care
student:

1. Over the next ten weeks, I will learn the definition,
   pronunciation, and spelling of 150 new medical terms.

2. Within the next month, I will attend one professional
   meeting and talk with two people I have not met
   before.

Making Goals Work for You

1. Set them! The main reason people do not achieve their
   goals is that they fail to set them in the first place.

2. Develop an action plan outlining the steps needed to
   reach them.

Continued

28 *Quick Review Section*

Goals

3. Set reasonable deadlines for each step.
4. Identify and locate any resources needed to carry out your action steps (examples: people, materials, classes, equipment, money).
5. Don't forget to include your goals when you plan your daily activities. (Goals are often put aside in the scramble to meet everyday obligations.)
6. Periodically evaluate your goals and progress and make necessary adjustments.
7. Visualize yourself achieving them.
8. Use affirmations.
9. Work on them even when you don't feel like it. (Especially then!)
10. Don't give up!

Developing a Plan

Goals work only if you work steadily toward achieving them. Let's look at an example of a goal plan for mastering the 150 medical terms.

Goal: Over the next ten weeks, I will learn the meaning, pronunciation, and correct spelling of 150 new medical terms.

Plan: Learn 15 new terms each week. Study terminology four hours a week using flash cards, the workbook, tapes, and self-quizzes. Quiz myself at the end of each week.

Deadline: 15 terms each week. Achieve goal of 150 words at the end of ten weeks on _____ (date).

Resources: Text and workbook; talk with instructors about suggestions for learning; check out tapes from the library; buy a medical dictionary.

Visualization: See self in class receiving 100% on the medical terminology test. See self using medical terms correctly when talking with a coworker on the job.

Affirmation: "I, _____ , am mastering medical language easily and on schedule."

From: Haroun, L. (2000). *Career Development for Health Professionals.* Phila.: W B Saunders, all of p. 44 (no top quote). Reprinted with permission.

BIG GOAL FORM

Completion Date
Exact or Approximate

Goal:

WHY this goal is worth the time & effort:

WHAT it will take (Action Steps):	DEADLINE for each
1.	
2.	
3.	
4.	
Other:	

RESOURCES I need:	Check when secured

VISUALIZATION/AFFIRMATION statement of goal:

Commitment Statement and Signature:
I accept this goal and agree to the action steps necessary to reach this
goal by _____ (date).

_____
Signature

Clip when complete
See other side for Notes ➡

Goals

BIG GOAL NOTES:

BIG GOAL FORM

Completion Date
Exact or Approximate

Goal:

WHY this goal is worth the time & effort:

WHAT it will take (Action Steps):	**DEADLINE** for each
1.	
2.	
3.	
4.	
Other:	

RESOURCES I need:	**Check** when secured

VISUALIZATION/AFFIRMATION statement of goal:

Commitment Statement and Signature:
I accept this goal and agree to the action steps necessary to reach this goal by _____ (date).

_____
Signature

Clip when complete
See other side for Notes ➡

Goals

BIG GOAL NOTES:

BIG GOAL FORM

Completion Date
Exact or Approximate

Goal:

WHY this goal is worth the time & effort:

WHAT it will take (Action Steps):	DEADLINE for each
1.	
2.	
3.	
4.	
Other:	

RESOURCES I need:	Check when secured

VISUALIZATION/AFFIRMATION statement of goal:

Commitment Statement and Signature:
I accept this goal and agree to the action steps necessary to reach this goal by _____ (date).

_____
Signature

Clip when complete
See other side for Notes ➡

BIG GOAL NOTES:

BIG GOAL FORM

Completion Date
Exact or Approximate

Goal:

WHY this goal is worth the time & effort:

WHAT it will take (Action Steps):	DEADLINE for each
1.	
2.	
3.	
4.	
Other:	

RESOURCES I need:	Check when secured

VISUALIZATION/AFFIRMATION statement of goal:

Commitment Statement and Signature:
I accept this goal and agree to the action steps necessary to reach this goal by _____ (date).

_____
Signature

Clip when complete
See other side for Notes ➡

BIG GOAL NOTES:

BIG GOAL FORM

Goal:

WHY this goal is worth the time & effort:

WHAT it will take (Action Steps):	**DEADLINE** for each
1.	
2.	
3.	
4.	
Other:	

RESOURCES I need:	**Check** when secured

VISUALIZATION/AFFIRMATION statement of goal:

Commitment Statement and Signature:
I accept this goal and agree to the action steps necessary to reach this
goal by _____ (date).

_____
Signature

Clip when complete
See other side for Notes ➡

BIG GOAL NOTES:

Abbreviations & Acronyms

Commonly Used Hospital Abbreviations

A

a	before
AA	Alcoholics Anonymous
aa	of each
AAROM	active assistive range of motion
abd.	abdomen
ABG	arterial blood gases
AC	alternating current; air conduction
a.c.	before meals
ACE	angiotensin-converting enzyme
ACh	acetylcholine
ACTH	adrenocorticotropic hormone
AD	right ear
ADA	American Diabetes Association; American Dental Association; Americans with Disabilities Act
ADH	antidiuretic hormone
ADL	activities of daily living
ad lib	as desired
a-fib	atrial fibrillation
A/G	albumin-globulin ratio
AHA	American Heart Association
AHF	antihemophilic factor
AIDS	acquired immunodeficiency syndrome
AK	above the knee
ALARA	as low as reasonably achievable (radiology)
ALL	acute lymphocytic leukemia
ALS	amyotrophic lateral sclerosis
AM	morning
AMA	against medical advice; American Medical Association
AMD	age-related macular degeneration
AMI	acute myocardial infarction
amp.	ampere
ant.	anterior

Continued

ANUG	acute necrotizing ulcerative gingivitis
AODM	adult-onset diabetes mellitus
AP	antepartum; anteroposterior
A & P	auscultation and percussion
A-P	anterior-posterior
APA	American Psychological Association
appt.	appointment
A/R	apical/radial
ARC	AIDS related complex
ARD	acute respiratory disease
ARF	acute renal failure
AROM	active range of motion; artificial rupture of membrane
ARROM	active resistive range of motion
AS	left ear
ASA	acetylsalicylic acid (aspirin)
ASAP	as soon as possible
ASCVD	arteriosclerotic cardiovascular disease
ASD	atrial septal defect
ASHD	arteriosclerotic heart disease
ASS	anterior superior spine
AST	aspartamine aminotransferase
Ast	astigmatism
AU	both ears; Angstrom unit
AV	artrioventricular; arteriovenous
av.	avoirdupois
A & W	alive and well
AWS	air water spray

B

Ba	barium
BAC	buccoaxiocervical
BBB	blood-brain barrier
BC/BS	Blue Cross/Blue Shield
BCP	birth control pill
BE	barium enema
BF	black female
b.i.d.	two times a day
BK	below the knee
BLE	bilateral lower extremity
BM	black male

Continued

bm	bowel movement
BMR	basal metabolic rate
BP	blood pressure
BPH	benign prostatic hypertrophy
BR	bathroom
BRP	bathroom privileges
BSA	body surface area
BSE	breast self-examination
BSP	Bromsulphalein
BUE	bilateral upper extremity
BUN	blood urea nitrogen
BVR	Bureau of Vocational Rehabilitation
BW	birth weight
bx	biopsy

C

C	centigrade
c	with
C(x)	C followed by a number indicates a specific cervical vertebra
CA	cancer; chronological age; cervicoaxillary
Ca	Calcium, cancer
CABG	coronary artery bypass graft
CABS	coronary artery bypass surgery
CAD	coronary artery disease
cap.	capsule
CAT	computerized axial tomography
CBC	complete blood count
CC	chief complaint
cc	cubic centimeter
CCU	Coronary Care Unit
CEJ	cementoenamel junction
CF	cystic fibrosis
CFIDS	chronic fatigue immune deficiency syndrome
CFT	complement fixation test
CH	crown-heel measurement
CHD	coronary heart disease
CHF	congestive heart failure
CHO	carbohydrate
cm	centimeter
CML	chronic myelogenous leukemia

Continued

CMV	cytomegalovirus
CNS	central nervous system
CO_2	carbon dioxide
C/O	complains of
col. ct.	colony count
comp.	compound
conc.	concentrated
COPD	chronic obstructive pulmonary disease
CP	cerebral palsy
CPD	cephalopelvic disproportion
CPK	creatine phosphokinase
CPR	cardiopulmonary resuscitation
CR	crown-rump length
CS	cesarean section
C & S	culture and sensitivity
CSF	cerebrospinal fluid
CT	computed tomography
CTS	carpal tunnel syndrome
CV	cardiovascular
CVA	cerebral vascular accident
CVD	cerebrovascular disease; cardiovascular disease
CVP	central venous pressure

D

DC	direct current
d.c.	discontinue
D&C	dilatation and currettage
D&E	dilation and evacuation
dg	decigram
DIC	disseminated intravascular coagulation
dil.	dilute
DJD	degenerative joint disease
DKA	diabetic ketoacidosis
dl	deciliter
DM	diabetes mellitus
DNA	deoxyribonucleic acid
DOA	dead on arrival; date of admission
DOB	date of birth
DOE	dyspnea on exertion
DPT	diphtheria, pertussis, tetanus
dr.	dram

Continued

dsg.	dressing
DTR	deep tendon reflex
DTs	delirium tremens
DVT	deep vein thrombosis
Dx	diagnosis

E

ECF	extended care facility
ECG	electrocardiogram
ECR	emergency chemical restraint
ECT	electroconvulsive therapy
ED	effective dose; erythema dose
EDC	estimated date of confinement
EDD	estimated date of delivery
EEG	electroencephalogram
EENT	eyes, ears, nose, and throat
EKG	electrocardiogram
EMG	electromyogram
EMS	emergency medical services
ENT	ears, nose, and throat
EOM	extraocular movement
ER	emergency room
ERG	electroretinogram
ESR	erythrocyte sedimentation rate
EST	electroshock therapy
ETOH	ethanol (ethyl alcohol)

F

F	Fahrenheit
FANA	fluorescent antinuclear antibody test
FBS	fasting blood sugar
FD	fatal dose; focal distance
FDA	Food and Drug Administration
Fe	iron
FEV	forced expiratory volume
FFA	free fatty acids
FH	family history
FHR	fetal heart rate
Fl	fluid
fld	fluid
FM	fine motor
FSH	follicle stimulating hormone
ft	foot

Continued

Abbreviations

FTND	full term normal delivery
FUO	fever of unknown origin
FWB	full weight bearing
Fx	fracture

G

G	gravida
GA	gingivoaxial
gal.	gallon
GB	gallbladder
GBS	gallbladder series
GC	gonococcus; gonorrhea
GFR	glomerular filtration rate
GG	gamma globulin
GI	gastrointestinal
GLA	gingivolinguoaxial
GM	gross motor
gm	gram
GP	general practitioner
gr.	grain
GSW	gunshot wound
GTT	glucose tolerance test
gtt.	drops
GU	genitourinary
GVHD	graft versus host disease
gyn	gynecology

H

Hb	hemoglobin
HBP	high blood pressure
HCG	human chorionic gonadotropin
hct.	hematocrit
HCTZ	hydrochlorothiazide
HD	hearing distance
HDL	high-density lipoprotein
HEENT	head, eye, ear, nose, and throat
Hg	mercury
Hgb	hemoglobin
H & H	hemoglobin and hematocrit
HHA	home health aide
HHNK	hyperglycemic, hyperosmolar nonketotic coma
HIV	human immunodeficiency virus

Continued

H_2O	water
H_2O_2	hydrogen peroxide
H & P	history and physical
HPI	history of present illness
HPV	high-power view
hs	hour of sleep
H-S	hepato-spleno
HSV	herpes simplex virus
HT	hypertension
Ht	total hyperopia
HTN	hypertension
HVD	hypertensive vascular disease
Hx	history
Hy	hyperopia
hyp.	hypodermic

I

I	iodine
IA	intra-arterial
IB	inclusion body
IBD	ideal body weight
ICP	intracranial pressure
ICS	intercostal space
ICU	Intensive Care Unit
I & D	incision and drainage
IDDM	insulin dependent diabetes mellitus
IM	intramuscular
inf.	infusion
inj.	injection
I & O	intake and output
IOP	intraocular pressure
IPPB	intermittent positive pressure breathing
IQ	intelligence quotient
ITP	idiopathic thrombocytopenic purpura
IU	international unit
IUD	intrauterine device
IV	intravenous
IVP	intravenous pyelogram
IVU	intravenous urogram

J

jt.	joint

Continued

K

K	potassium
KCl	potassium chloride
kg	kilogram
KOH	potassium hydroxide
KUB	kidney, ureters, and bladder
kv	kilovolt
KVO	keep vein open
kw	kilowatt

L

L	left, liter
L(x)	L followed by a number indicates a specific lumbar vertebra
l	liter
L & A	light and accommodation
lat.	lateral
lb	pound
LBP	low back pain
LCM	left costal margin
LD	lethal dose; light difference
LDL	low density lipoprotein
LE	lupus erythematosus; lower extremity
LGA	large for gestational age
LH	luteinizing hormone
LIF	left iliac fossa
lig.	ligament
Liq.	liquid
LLE	left lower extremity
LLL	left lower lobe
LLQ	left lower quadrant
LMP	last menstrual period
LOA	left occipitoposterior
LOT	left occipitotransverse
LP	lumbar puncture
LPV	low-power view
LUE	left upper extremity
LUL	left upper lobe
LUQ	left upper quadrant
LVH	left ventricular hypertrophy
L & W	living and well

Continued

M

m	meter
MAP	mean arterial pressure
MBD	minimal brain dysfunction
mc	millicurie
mcg	microgram
MCH	mean corpuscular hemoglobin
MCHC	mean corpuscular hemoglobin concentration
mCi	millicurie
MCL	mid-clavicular line
MCV	mean corpuscular volume
MD	muscular dystrophy; medical doctor
MED	minimal effective dose; minimal erythema dose
mEq	milliequivalents
mEq/L	milliequivalents per liter
Mg	magnesium
mg	milligram
MH	mental health; marital history
MI	myocardial infarction
min	minim; minute
ml	milliliter
mM	millimole
MMT	manual muscle test
mol. wt.	molecular weight
MOM	milk of magnes~a
MOPP	Mustargen, Oncovin, procarbazine, prednisone
MPV	medium-power view
MRI	magnetic resonance imaging
MS	mitral stenosis; multiple sclerosis
MSL	mid-sternal line
MVR	mitral valve replacement
MW	molecular weight
My	myopia

N

Na	sodium
N/A	not applicable
NaCl	sodium chloride
NAD	no acute distress; no appreciable disease
NAS	no added salt

Continued

NB	newborn
neg.	negative
NG	nasogastric
NIDDM	non–insulin dependent diabetes mellitus
NIH	National Institutes of Health
NKA	no known allergies
NMR	nuclear magnetic resonance
NPO	nothing by mouth
NSAID	nonsteroidal anti-inflammatory drug
NSR	normal sinus rhythm
NSS	normal saline solution
NSVD	normal spontaneous vaginal delivery
N & V	nausea and vomiting
NWB	non–weight bearing
NYD	not yet diagnosed

O

O_2	oxygen
OA	osteoarthritis; occipitoanterior
OB	obstetrics
OBS	organic brain syndrome
OC	oral contraceptive
OD	right eye
od	daily
O/F	oxidation fermentation
OL	left eye
OOB	out of bed
OP	occipitoposterior
OPD	outpatient department
OPV	oral polio vaccine
OR	operating room
ORIF	open reduction internal fixation
OS	left eye
OSHA	Occupational Safety and Health Administration
OT	occupational therapy
OTC	over the counter
OU	both eyes
oz	ounce

P

P	pulse
p	after

Continued

PA	pernicious anemia; posterior-anterior
P&A	percussion and auscultation
PAC	premature atrial contractions
PAP	Papanicolaou (test)
para	number of pregnancies
PBI	protein-bound iodine
p.c.	after meals
pct.	per cent
PCV	packed cell volume
PD	pupillary distance
PDA	patent ductus arteriosus
PDR	Physicians' Desk Reference
PE	physical examination
P.E.	physical examination; pulmonary emboli
PEG	percutaneous esophagogastrectomy; pneumoencephalogram
PERLA	pupils equal, react to light and accommodation
PERRLA	pupils equal, round, react to light and accommodation
PET	positron emission tomography
PH	past history
Pl	present illness
PID	pelvic inflammatory disease
PIH	pregnancy-induced hypertension
PKU	phenylketonuria
PM	afternoon; evening; postmortem
P.M.	perceptual motor
PMH	past medical history
PMI	point of maximal impulse
PMP	previous menstrual period
PMS	premenstrual syndrome
PND	paroxysmal nocturnal dyspnea
p.o.	by mouth
P.O.R.	problem-oriented record
pp	postpartum; postprandial
PPD	purified protein derivative (tuberculin)
ppm	parts per million
pr	per rectum
PRE	progressive resistive exercise
prn	as needed
PROM	passive range of motion

Abbreviations

Continued

pro time	prothrombin time
PSS	physiologic saline solution
pt.	patient; pint
PT	prothrombin time; physical therapy
PTA	prior to admission; plasma thromboplastin antecedent
PTT	partial thromboplastin time
PVC	premature ventricular contraction
PVD	peripheral vascular disease
PWB	partial weight bearing

Q

q	every
q.d.	every day
qh	every hour
q.n.s.	quantity not sufficient
q.o.d.	every other day
q.s.	quantity sufficient
qt.	quart

R

RA	rheumatoid arthritis
rad	radiation absorbed dose
RAI	radioactive iodine
RAIU	radioactive iodine uptake
RBC	red blood count
RDA	recommended daily allowance
RDS	respiratory distress syndrome
Rh	Rhesus factor
RHD	rheumatic heart disease
RLE	right lower extremity
RLL	right lower lobe
RLQ	right lower quadrant
RML	right middle lobe
r/o	rule out
ROA	right occipitoanterior
ROM	range of motion
ROP	right occipitoposterior
ROS	review of symptoms
ROT	right occipitotransverse
RPM; rpm	revolutions per minute
RPRC	rapid plasma reagin card test (for syphilis)

Continued

RR	respiratory rate
R/T	related to
rt.	right
RUE	right upper extremity
RUL	right upper lobe
RUQ	right upper quadrant
Rx	treatment, therapy, prescription

S

s	without
sc.	subcutaneous
SGA	small for gestational age
SGOT	serum glutamic-oxaloacetic transaminase
SGPT	serum glutamic pyruvate transaminase
SH	social history; serum hepatitis
sib.	sibling
SID	sudden infant death syndrome
SIDS	sudden infant death syndrome
sig.	label
sl	sublingual
SLE	systemic lupus erythematosus
SNF	skilled nursing facility
S.O.A.P.	subjective, objective, assessment, plan
SOB	shortness of breath
s/p	status post
SPF	sun protection factor
sp.gr.	specific gravity
spt.	spirit
ss	one half
SSE	soap suds enema
SSS	sick sinus syndrome
S & Sx	signs and symptoms
stat	immediately
STD	sexually transmitted disease
STS	serologic test for syphilis
sub. q.	subcutaneous
SUID	sudden unexplained infant death
SVD	spontaneous vaginal delivery
SVT	supraventricular tachycardia
Sx	symptoms
sym.	symmetrical
syr.	syrup

Abbreviations

Continued

T

T.	tablespoon; temperature
T(x)	T followed by a number indicates a specific thoracic vertebra
T & A	tonsillectomy and adenoidectomy
tab.	tablet
TAH	total abdominal hysterectomy
TAH-BSO	total abdominal hysterectomy-bilateral salpingo-oophorectomy
TAT	tetanus antitoxin
TB	tuberculosis
tbsp.	tablespoon
TIA	transient ischemic attack
t.i.d.	three times a day
TNTC	too numerous to count
T.O.	telephone order
TPN	total parenteral nutrition
TPR	temperature, pulse, respiration
tr.	trace; tincture
tinct	tincture
tsp.	teaspoon
TUR	transurethral resection
TURP	transurethral resection of the prostate

U

U	unit
UA	urinalysis
UE	upper extremity
UHF	ultrahigh frequency
ung.	ointment
UQ	upper quadrant
URI	upper respiratory infection
USP	United States Pharmacopeia
UTI	urinary tract infection
UV	ultraviolet

V

v	volt
VA	Veterans Administration; visual acuity
VC	vital capacity
VD	venereal disease
VDA	visual discriminatory acuity

Continued

Vfib	ventricular fibrillation
VHD	valvular heart disease
VLDL	very-low-density lipoprotein
V.O.	verbal order
v s.	vital signs
VSD	ventricular septal defect
VT	ventricular tachycardia

W

W	watt
WBAT	weight bearing as tolerated
WBC	white blood count
w.b.c.	white blood count
w/c	wheelchair
WD	well-developed
WDWN	well-developed, well-nourished
WF	white female
wk.	week
WL	wavelength
WM	white male
WN	well-nourished
WNL	within normal limits
wo	without
wt.	weight

X

| x | times |
| x-ray | roentgen ray |

Most hospitals, commmunity health agencies, and other clinical facilities have a list of approved abbreviations to be used in patient records. The abbreviations listed below are often used when charting and will assist in the interpretation of patient records, but they should not be utilized on the record unless they are on the approved list for the clinical site.

The following are a few abbreviations used to refer to health care providers and insurers:

BC/BS—Blue Cross, Blue Shield, a national insurance organization that makes payments for a wide variety of health care services for its subscribers. Frequently referred to as the "Blues."

Continued

Abbreviations

CHAMPUS—the civilian health and medical program of the uniformed services, a program that is administered by the Department of Defense. CHAMPUS pays for health care services to active and retired members of the uniformed services and reimburses providers for the health care of the dependents of eligible personnel.

HMO—health maintenance organization, an organization that provides preventive health services as well as medical, hospital, and emergency care for members. There is a fee, paid in advance, to belong to a HMO.

IPA—independent practice association, a type of health maintenance organization in which the organization contracts with physicians who see patients in their own offices, rather than at a specific location designated as an HMO. The physicians are reimbursed by the HMO.

Medicare, Part A—Title XVIII of Health Insurance for the Aged of the Social Security Act. Medicare, Part A reimburses the hospital for services provided to eligible patients.

Medicare, Part B—Title XVIII of Health Insurance for the Aged of the Social Security Act. Medicare, Part B reimburses physicians for services provided to eligible patients. This insurance is provided to eligible citizens only when a supplementary payment is made.

PPO—Preferred Provider Organization, an association of hospitals, physicians, and agencies that provides health care to a specific group of individuals at agreed-upon rates.

From: Miller/Keane: Encyclopedia & Dictionary of Medicine, Nursing, & Allied Health (6th ed.). Philadelphia: WB Saunders, p.1867-1872. Reprinted with permission.

Acronyms for Selected Health Care Organizations, Associations, and Agencies

AAAA	American Academy of Anesthesiologist's Assistants
AAATP	Association for Anesthesiologist's Assistants Training Program
AAB	American Association of Bioanalysts
AABB	American Association of Blood Banks
AACA	American Association of Clinical Anatomists
AACAHPO	American Association of Certified Allied Health Personnel in Ophthalmology
AACC	American Association for Clinical Chemistry
AACCN	American Association of Critical Care Nurses
AACN	American Association of Colleges of Nursing
AADS	American Association of Dental Schools
AAFP	American Academy of Family Physicians
AAHA	American Academy of Health Administration
AAHC	Association of Academic Health Centers
AAHE	Association for the Advancement of Health Education
AAHP	American Association of Hospital Planners
AAHPER	American Association for Health, Physical Education, and Recreation
AAMA	American Association of Medical Assistants
AAMC	Association of American Medical Colleges
AAMI	Association for the Advancement of Medical Instrumentation
AAMT	American Association for Music Therapy
AAN	American Academy of Neurology
AANA	American Association of Nurse Anesthetists

Continued

Abbreviations

AAO	American Association of Ophthalmology
AAO	American Association of Orthodontists
AAOHN	American Association of Occupational Health Nurses
AAP	American Academy of Pediatrics
AAPA	American Academy of Physicians Assistants
AAPMR	American Academy of Physical Medicine and Rehabilitation
AARC	American Association for Respiratory Care
AART	American Association for Rehabilitation Therapy
AATA	American Art Therapy Association
AATS	American Association for Thoracic Surgery
ABCP	American Board of Cardiovascular Perfusion
ABNF	Association of Black Nursing Faculty in Higher Education
ACC	American College of Cardiology
ACCP	American College of Chest Physicians
ACEN	Academy of Chief Executive Nurses (Canada)
ACEP	American College of Emergency Physicians
ACHA	American College of Hospital Administrators
ACNM	American College of Nurse-Midwives
ACP	American College of Physicians
ACR	American College of Radiology
ACS	American College of Surgeons
ACTA	American Cardiovascular Technologists Association
ACTA	American Corrective Therapy Association
ADA	American Dental Association
ADA	American Dietetic Association
ADAA	American Dental Assistants Association
ADHA	American Dental Hygienists' Association
ADTA	American Dance Therapy Association
AES	American Electroencephalographic Society

Continued

AHA	American Hospital Association
AHIMA	American Health Information Management Association
AHPA	American Health Planning Association
AIBS	American Institute of Biological Sciences
AIHA	American Industrial Hygiene Association
AIUM	American Institute of Ultrasound in Medicine
AMA	American Medical Association
AMEA	American Medical Electroencephalographic Association
AMI	Association of Medical Illustrators
AmSECT	American Society of Extra-Corporeal Technology
AMT	American Medical Technologists
ANA	American Nurses Association
ANF	American Nurses Foundation
ANNA	American Nephrology Nurses' Association
ANRC	American National Red Cross
AOA	American Optometric Association
AOA	American Osteopathic Association
AONE	American Organization of Nurse Executives
AORN	Association of Operating Room Nurses
AOTA	American Occupational Therapy Association
APA	American Podiatry Association
APA	American Psychiatric Association
APA	American Psychological Association
APAP	Association of Physician Assistants Programs
APHA	American Public Health Association
APIC	Association of Practitioners in Infection Control
APTA	American Physical Therapy Association
ARCA	American Rehabilitation Counseling Association
ARN	Association of Rehabilitation Nurses
ASA	American Society of Anesthesiologists
ASAHP	American Society of Allied Health Professionals

Continued

ASC	American Society of Cytotechnology
ASCP	American Society of Clinical Pathologists
ASE	American Society of Echocardiography
ASET	American Society of Electroencephalographic Technologists
ASHA	American Speech and Hearing Association
ASIA	American Spinal Injury Association
ASIM	American Society of Internal Medicine
ASM	American Society of Microbiology
ASMT	American Society for Medical Technology
ASNSA	American Society of Nursing Service Administrators
ASPAN	American Association of Post Anesthesia Nurses
ASPH	Association of Schools of Public Health
ASRT	American Society of Radiologic Technologists
AST	Association of Surgical Technologists
ASUTS	American Society of Ultrasound Technical Specialists
ATS	American Thoracic Society
AUPHA	Association of University Programs in Health Administration
AVA	American Vocational Association
AVMA	American Veterinary Medical Association
CAP	College of American Pathologists
CAHEA (AMA)	Committee on Allied Health Education and Accreditation
CCHFA	Canadian Council of Health Facilities Accreditation
CCHSE	Canadian Council of Health Service Executives
CDC	Centers for Disease Control and Prevention
CGFNS	Commission on Graduates of Foreign Nursing Schools
CGNA	Canadian Gerontological Nursing Association
CME (AMA)	Council on Medical Education of the American Medical Association

Continued

CNA	Canadian Nurses Association
COEAMRA	Council on Education of the American Medical Record Association
DHHS	Department of Health and Human Services
ENA	Emergency Nurses Association
FDA	Food and Drug Administration
HCFA	Health Care Financing Administration
HRA	Health Resources Administration
HSCA	Health Sciences Communications Association
HSRA	Health Services and Resources Administration
IAET	International Association for Enterostomal Therapy
ISCV	International Society for Cardiovascular Surgery
JCAHO	Joint Commission on the Accreditation of Healthcare Organizations
JCAHPO	Joint Commission on Allied Health Personnel in Ophthalmology
MLA	Medical Library Association
NMCLS	National Accrediting Agency for Clinical Laboratory Science
NAACOG	Nurses Association of the American Association of Obstetrics and Gynecology
NACA	National Advisory Council on Aging—Canadian
NACT	National Alliance of Cardiovascular Technologists
NADONA/LTC	National Association of Directors of Nursing Administration in Long Term Care
NAEMT	National Association of Emergency Medical Technicians
NAHC	National Association of Home Care
NAHM	National Association for Mental Health
NAHSR	National Association of Human Services Technologists
NAMT	National Association for Music Therapy
NANDA	North American Nursing Diagnosis Association

Abbreviations

Continued

NANPHR	National Association of Nurse Practitioners in Reproductive Health
NANT	National Association of Nephrology Technologists
NAPNES	National Association for Practical Nurse Education and Services
NARF	National Association of Rehabilitation Facilities
NASW	National Association of Social Workers
NATTS	National Association of Trade and Technical Schools
NCEHPHP	National Council on the Education of Health Professionals in Health Promotion
NCRE	National Council on Rehabilitation Education
NEHA	National Environmental Health Education
NFLPN	National Federation of Licensed Practical Nurses
NHC	National Health Council
NIH	National Institutes of Health
NIOSH	National Institute of Occupational Safety and Health
NKF	National Kidney Foundation
NLN	National League for Nursing
NNBA	National Nurses in Business Association
NRCA	National Rehabilitation Counseling Association
NREMT	National Registry of Emergency Medical Technicians
NSCPT	National Society for Cardiopulmonary Technology
NSH	National Society for Histotechnology
NSNA	National Student Nurses Association
NTRS	National Therapeutic Recreation Society
OAA	Opticians Association of America
ONS	Oncology Nurses Association
SAAABB	Subcommittee on Accreditation of the American Association of Blood Banks
SDMS	Society of Diagnostic Medical Sonographers
SNIVT	Society of Non-Invasive Vascular Technology

Continued

SNM	Society of Nuclear Medicine
SNM-TS	Society for Nuclear Medicine—Technologists Section
SPHE	Society of Public Health Educators
STS	Society of Thoracic Surgeons
SVS	Society for Vascular Surgery
TAANA	American Association of Nurse Attorneys
USPHS	United States Public Health Services
VA	Veterans Affairs
WHO	World Health Organization

Abbreviations

From: Miller/Keane: Encyclopedia & Dictionary of Medicine, Nursing, & Allied Health (6th ed.). Philadelphia: WB Saunders, p.1889-1891. Reprinted with permission.

Professional Designations for Health Care Providers

Degrees, certifications, memberships and other initials that precede or follow the names of health care providers often provide helpful information regarding their area of expertise and level of practice.The following list identifies commonly used designations in English speaking countries, particularly the United States and Canada.

ANP	Adult Nurse Practitioner
ARNP	Advanced Registered Nurse Practitioner
BA	Bachelor of Arts
BB(ASCP)	Technologist in Blood Banking certified by The American Society of Clinical Pathologists
BDentSci	Bachelor of Dental Science
BDS	Bachelor of Dental Surgery
BDSc	Bachelor of Dental Science
BHS	Bachelor of Health Science
BHyg	Bachelor of Hygiene
BM	Bachelor of Medicine
BMed	Bachelor of Medicine
BMedBiol	Bachelor of Medical Biology
BMedSci	Bachelor of Medical Science
BMic	Bachelor of Microbiology
BMS	Bachelor of Medical Science
BMT	Bachelor of Medical Technology
BO	Bachelor of Osteopathy
BP	Bachelor of Pharmacy
BPH	Bachelor of Public Health
BPharm	Bachelor of Pharmacy
BPHEng	Bachelor of Public Health Engineering
BPHN	Bachelor of Public Health Nursing
BPsTh	Bachelor of Psychotherapy
BS	Bachelor of Science
BSM	Bachelor of Science in Medicine
BSN	Bachelor of Science in Nursing
BSPh	Bachelor of Science in Pharmacy
BSS	Bachelor of Sanitary Science
BVMS	Bachelor of Veterinary Medicine and Science

Continued

BVSc	Bachelor of Veterinary Science
CALN	Clinical Administrative Liaison Nurse
C(ASCP)	Technologist in Chemistry certified by the American Society of Clinical Pathologists
CB	Bachelor of Surgery
CCRN	Critical Care Registered Nurse
CDA	Certified Dental Assistant
CEN	Certificate for Emergency Nursing
CEO	Chief Executive Officer
ChB	Bachelor of Surgery
ChD	Doctor of Surgery
ChM	Master of Surgery
CIH	Certificate in Industrial Health
CLA	Certified Laboratory Assistant
CLS	Clinical Laboratory Scientist
CLS(NCA)	Clinical Laboratory Scientist certified by the National Certification Agency for Medical Laboratory Personnel
CLT	Certified Laboratory Technician; Clinical Laboratory Technician
CLT(NCA)	Laboratory Technician certified by the National Certification Agency for Medical Laboratory Personnel
CM	Master of Surgery
CMA	Certified Medical Assistant
CMO	Chief Medical Officer
CNM	Certified Nurse Midwife
CNMT	Certified Nuclear Medicine Technologist
CNP	Community Nurse Practitioner
CNS	Clinical Nurse Specialist
CORN	Certified Operating Room Nurse
COTA	Certified Occupational Therapy Assistant
CPAN	Certified Post Anesthesia Nurse
CPH	Certificate in Public Health
CPNP	Certified Pediatric Nurse Practitioner
CRNA	Certified Registered Nurse Anesthetist
CRRN	Certified Registered Rehabilitation Nurse
CRTT	Certified Respiratory Therapy Technician
CT(ASCP)	Cytotechnologist certified by the American Society of Clinical Pathologists
CURN	Certified Urological Registered Nurse
CVO	Chief Veterinary Officer

Continued

Abbreviations

DA	Dental Assistant; Diploma in Anesthetics
DC	Doctor of Chiropractic
DCH	Diploma in Child Health
DCh	Doctor of Surgery
DChO	Doctor of Ophthalmic Surgery
DCM	Doctor of Comparative Medicine
DCOG	Diploma of the College of Obstetricians and Gynaecologists
DCP	Diploma in Clinical Pathology; Diploma in Clinical Psychology
DDH	Diploma in Dental Health
DDM	Doctor of Dental Medicine; Diploma in Dermatologic Medicine
DDO	Diploma in Dental Orthopaedics
DDR	Diploma in Diagnostic Radiology
DDS	Doctor of Dental Surgery
DDSc	Doctor of Dental Science
DFHom	Diploma of the Faculty of Homeopathy
DHg	Doctor of Hygiene
DHy	Doctor of Hygiene
DHyg	Doctor of Hygiene
Dip	Diplomate
DipBact	Diploma in Bacteriology
DipChem	Diploma in Chemistry
DipClinPath	Diploma in Clinical Pathology
DipMicrobiol	Diploma in Microbiology
DipSocMed	Diploma in Social Medicine
DLM(ASCP)	Diplomate in Laboratory Management
DMD	Doctor of Dental Medicine
DMT	Doctor of Medical Technology
DMV	Doctor of Veterinary Medicine
DN	Doctor of Nursing
DNE	Doctor of Nursing Education
DNS	Doctor of Nursing Science
DNSc	Doctor of Nursing Science
DO	Doctor of Osteopathy; Doctor of Optometry; Doctor of Ophthalmology
DON	Director of Nursing
DOS	Doctor of Ocular Science; Doctor of Optical Science
DP	Doctor of Pharmacy, Doctor of Podiatry

Continued

DPH	Doctor of Public Hygiene; Doctor of Public Health
DPhC	Doctor of Pharmaceutical Chemistry
DPHN	Doctor of Public Health Nursing
DPhys	Diploma in Physiotherapy
DPM	Doctor of Podiatric Medicine, Doctor of Physical Medicine; Doctor of Preventive Medicine; Doctor of Psychiatric Medicine
Dr	Doctor
DrHyg	Doctor of Hygiene
DrMed	Doctor of Medicine
DrPH	Doctor of Public Health; Doctor of Public Hygiene
DSc	Doctor of Science
DSE	Doctor of Sanitary Engineering
DSIM	Doctor of Science in Industrial Medicine
DSSc	Diploma in Sanitary Science
DVM	Doctor of Veterinary Medicine
DVMS	Doctor of Veterinary Medicine and Surgery
DVR	Doctor of Veterinary Radiology
DVS	Doctor of Veterinary Science; Doctor of Veterinary Medicine
DVSc	Doctor of Veterinary Science
Ed.D.	Doctor of Education
ET	Enterostomal Therapist
FAAN	Fellow of the American Academy of Nurses
FACA	Fellow of the American College of Anesthetists; Fellow of the American College of Angiology, Fellow of the American College of Apothecaries
FACAI	Fellow of the American College of Allergists
FACC	Fellow of the American College of Cardiologists
FACCP	Fellow of the American College of Chest Physicians
FACD	Fellow of the American College of Dentists
FACFP	Fellow of the American College of Family Physicians

Continued

Abbreviations

FACG	Fellow of the American College of Gastroenterology
FACHA	Fellow of the American College of Health Administrators
FACOG	Fellow of the American College of Obstetricians and Gynecologists
FACP	Fellow of the American College of Physicians
FACPM	Fellow of the American College of Preventive Medicine
FACS	Fellow of the American College of Surgeons
FACSM	Fellow of the American College of Sports Medicine
FAMA	Fellow of the American Medicine Association
FAOTA	Fellow of the American Occupational Therapy Association
FAPA	Fellow of the American Psychiatric Association
FAPHA	Fellow of the American Public Health Association
FBPsS	Fellow of the British Psychological Association
FCAP	Fellow of the College of American Pathologists
FCMS	Fellow of the College of Medicine and Surgery
FCO	Fellow of the College of Osteopathy
FCPS	Fellow of the College of Physicians and Surgeons
FCSP	Fellow of the Chartered Society of Physiotherapy
FCST	Fellow of the College of Speech Therapists
FDS	Fellow in Dental Surgery
FDSRCSEng	Fellow in Dental Surgery of the Royal College of Surgeons of England
FFA	Fellow of the Faculty of Anesthetists
FFCM	Fellow of the Faculty of Community Medicine
FFD	Fellow in the Faculty of Dentistry

Continued

FFOM	Fellow of the Faculty of Occupational Medicine
FFR	Fellow of the Faculty of Radiologists
FIB	Fellow in the Institute of Biology
FICD	Fellow of the Institute of Canadian Dentists; Fellow of the International College of Dentists
FIMLT	Fellow of the Institute of Medical Laboratory Technology
FNP	Family Nurse Practitioner
FPS	Fellow of the Pathological Society
FRCD	Fellow of the Royal College of Dentists
FRCGP	Fellow of the Royal College of General Practitioners
FRCOG	Fellow of the Royal College of Obstetricians and Gynaecologists
FRCP	Fellow of the Royal College of Physicians
FRCPath	Fellow of the Royal College of Pathologists
FRCP(C)	Fellow of the Royal College of Physicians of Canada
FRCS	Fellow of the Royal College of Surgeons
FRCS(C)	Fellow of the Royal College of Surgeons of Canada
GNP	Gerontological Nurse Practitioner
H(ASCP)	Technologist in Hematology certified by the American Society of Clinical Pathologists
HT(ASCP)	Histologic Technician certified by the American Society of Clinical Pathologists
HTL(ASCP)	Histotechnologist certified by the American Society of Clinical Pathologists
TI(ASCP)	Technologist in Immunology certified by the American Society of Clinical Pathologists
LMCC	Licentiate of the Medical Council of Canada
LMRCP	Licentiate in Midwifery of the Royal College of Physicians
LPN	Licensed Practical Nurse
LVN	Licensed Vocational Nurse
MA	Master of Arts
M(ASCP)	Technologist in Microbiology certified by the American Society of Clinical Pathologists

Continued

MB	Bachelor of Medicine
MC	Mastery of Surgery
MCPS	Member of the College of Physicians and Surgeons
MD	Doctor of Medicine
MDentSc	Master of Dental Science
MDS	Master of Dental Surgery
MLT	Medical Laboratory Technician
MLT(ASCP)	Medical Laboratory Technician certified by the American Society of Clinical Pathologists
MMS	Master of Medical Science
MMSA	Master of Midwifery
MPH	Master of Public Health
MPharm	Master of Pharmacy
MRad	Master of Radiology
MRL	Medical Records Librarian
MS	Master of Science; Master of Surgery
MSB	Master of Science in Bacteriology
MSc	Master of Science
MScD	Master of Dental Science
MScN	Master of Science in Nursing
MSN	Master of Science in Nursing
MSPH	Master of Science in Public Health
MSPhar	Master of Science in Pharmacy
MSSc	Master of Sanitary Science
MSW	Master of Social Work; Medical Social Worker
MT	Medical Technologist
MT(ASCP)	Medical Technologist certified by the American Society of Clinical Pathologists
MVD	Doctor of Veterinary Medicine
ND	Doctor of Nursing
NM(ASCP)	Technologist in Nuclear Medicine certified by the American Society of Clinical Pathologists
NP	Nurse Practitioner
OD	Doctor of Optometry
ONC	Orthopedic Nursing Certificate
OT	Occupational Therapist
OTL	Occupational Therapist, Licensed
OTR	Occupational Therapist, Registered
OTReg	Occupational Therapist, Registered

Continued

PA   Physician's Assistant
PBT(ASCP)   Phlebotomy Technician certified by the
                  American Society of Clinical Pathologists
PCP   Primary Care Physician
PD   Doctor of Pharmacy
Ph.D.   Doctor of Philosophy; Doctor of Pharmacy
PNP   Pediatric Nurse Practitioner
PT   Physical Therapist
RDA   Registered Dental Assistant
Reg   Registered
RHIA   Registered Health Information
                  Administrator
RHIT   Registered Health Information Technician
RMA   Registered Medical Assistant
RN   Registered Nurse
RNA   Registered Nurse Anesthetist
RN,C.   Registered Nurse Certified (used to
                  identify nurses certified by the American
                  Nurses Credentialing Center; areas of
                  practice are medical-surgical nurse,
                  gerontological nurse, psychiatric and
                  mental health nurse, pediatric nurse,
                  perinatal nurse, community health nurse,
                  school nurse, general nursing practice,
                  college health nurse, gerontologic nurse
                  practitioner, pediatric nurse practitioner,
                  adult nurse practitioner, family nurse
                  practitioner, and school nurse practitioner)
RN,C.N.A.   Registered Nurse, Certified in Nursing
                  Administration
RN, CNNA   Registered Nurse, Certified in Nursing
                  Administration, Advanced
RN,C.S.   Registered Nurse, Certified Specialist
                  (used to identify nurses certified by the
                  American Nurses Credentialing Center;
                  this certification recognizes clinical
                  specialists in the following areas:
                  gerontological nursing, medical surgical
                  nursing, adult psychiatric and mental
                  health nursing, child and adolescent
                  psychiatric and mental health nursing,
                  and community health nursing)

Continued

Abbreviations

RPh	Registered Pharmacist
RPT	Registered Physical Therapist
RRL	Registered Record Librarian
RRT	Registered Respiratory Therapist
RT	Radiologic Technologist; Respiratory Therapist
RT(N)	Nuclear Medicine Technologist
RT(R)	Technologist in Diagnostic Radiology
RTR	Registered Recreational Therapist
RT(T)	Radiation Therapy Technologist
SBB(ASCP)	Specialist in Blood Banking certified by the American Society of Clinical Pathologists
ScD	Doctor of Science
SCT(ASCP)	Specialist in Cytotechnology certified by the American Society of Clinical Pathologists
SNP	School Nurse Practitioner
SW	Social Worker

From: Miller/Keane: Encyclopedia & Dictionary of Medicine, Nursing, & Allied Health (6th ed.). Philadelphia: WB Saunders, p.1892-1895. Reprinted with permission.

Abbreviations

Anatomy Reference

Table of Bones, Listed by Regions of the Body

Region	Name	Total Number
Axial skeleton	Skull 21	
	(eight paired—16)	
	inferior nasal concha	
	lacrimal	
	maxilla	
	nasal	
	palatine	
	parietal	
	temporal	
	zygomatic	
	(five unpaired—5)	
	ethmoid	
	frontal	
	occipital	
	sphenoid	
	vomer	
	Ossicles of each ear 6	
	incus	
	malleus	
	stapes	
	Lower jaw	
	mandible 1	
	Neck	
	hyoid 1	
	Vertebral column 26	
	cervical vertebrae (7)	
	(atlas)	
	(axis)	
	thoracic vertebrae (12)	
	lumbar vertebrae (5)	
	sacrum (5 fused)	
	coccyx (4—5 fused)	
	Chest	
	sternum 1	
	ribs (12 pairs) 24	

Continued

Anatomy

Table of Bones, Listed by Regions of the Body *(continued)*

Region	Name	Total Number
Upper limb (×2) 64		
Shoulder	scapula	
	clavicle	
Upper arm	humerus	
Lower arm	radius	
	ulna	
Wrist	carpal (8)	
	(capitate)	
	(hamate)	
	(lunate)	
	(pisiform)	
	(scaphoid)	
	(trapezium)	
	(trapezoid)	
	(triquetral)	
Hand	metacarpal (5)	
Fingers	phalanges (14)	
Lower limb (×2) 62		
Pelvis	hip bone (1)	
	(ilium)	
	(ischium)	
	(pubis)	
Thigh	femur	
Knee	patella	
Leg	tibia	
	fibula	
Ankle	tarsal (7)	
	(calcaneus)	
	(cuboid)	
	(cuneiform, medial)	
	(cuneiform, intermediate)	
	(cuneiform, lateral)	
	(navicular)	
	(talus)	
Foot	metatarsal (5)	
Toes	phalanges (14)	

Anatomy

From: Miller/Keane: Encyclopedia & Dictionary of Medicine, Nursing, & Allied Health (6th ed.). Philadelphia: WB Saunders, p.218. Reprinted with permission.

Anatomy

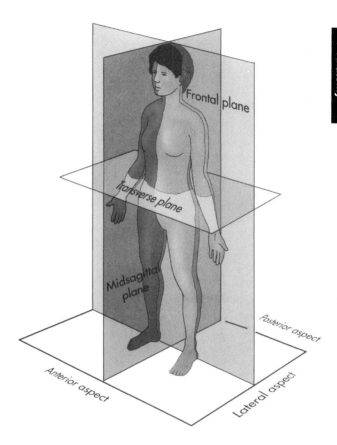

Frontal plane

Transverse plane

Midsagittal plane

Posterior aspect

Anterior aspect

Lateral aspect

Anatomic Position of the Body

From: Leonard, P. (2001) IM to acc. Building a Medical Vocabulary (5th ed.). St. Louis: WB Saunders, TM 1(Fig. 3-1 of text, p. 44). Reprinted with permission.

Anatomy

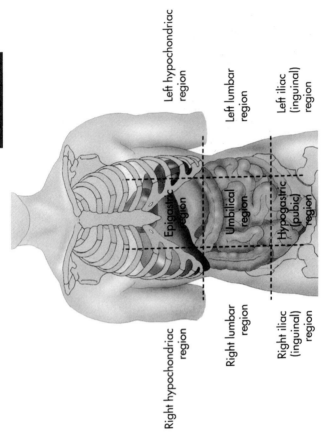

Right hypochondriac region

Left hypochondriac region

Epigastric region

Left lumbar region

Right lumbar region

Umbilical region

Left iliac (inguinal) region

Right iliac (inguinal) region

Hypogastric (pubic) region

Anatomic Regions of the Body

From: Leonard, P. (2001) IM to acc.
Building a Medical Vocabulary (5th ed.).
St. Louis: WB Saunders, TM 4 (Fig. 3-3b
of text, p. 50). Reprinted with permission.

Anatomy

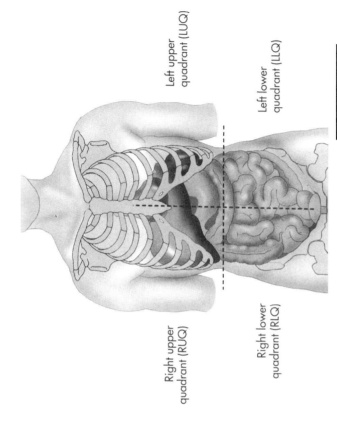

Left upper quadrant (LUQ)

Left lower quadrant (LLQ)

Right upper quadrant (RUQ)

Right lower quadrant (RLQ)

Quadrants of the Abdomen

From: Leonard, P. (2001) IM to acc.
Building a Medical Vocabulary (5th ed.).
St. Louis: WB Saunders, TM 3 (Fig. 3-3a
of text, p. 50). Reprinted with permission.

Anatomy

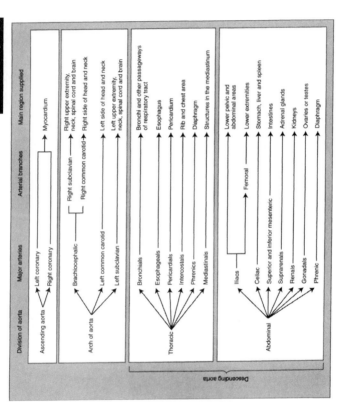

Aorta and Its Branches

From: Leonard. P. (2001) IM to acc.
Building a Medical Vocabulary (5th ed.).
St. Louis: WB Saunders, TM 16 (Fig. 5-7
of text, p. 121). Reprinted with permission.

Anatomy

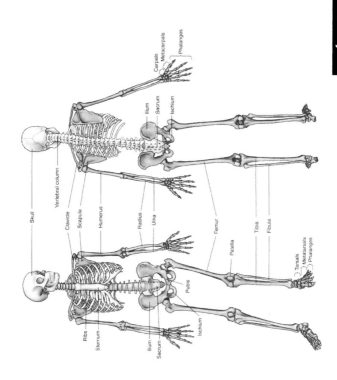

Human Skeleton with Major Bones

From: Leonard, P. (2001) IM to acc.
Building a Medical Vocabulary (5th ed.).
St. Louis: WB Saunders, TM 35 (Fig. 10-3
of text, p. 342). Reprinted with permission.

Lab Test Reference Values

Reference Values in Hematology

	Conventional Units	SI Units
Acid hemolysis test (Ham)	No hemolysis	No hemolysis
Alkaline phosphatase, leukocyte	Total score 14–100	Total score 14–100
Cell counts		
Erythrocytes		
Males	4.6–6.2 million/mm³	4.6–6.2 × 10¹²/L
Females	4.2–5.4 million/mm³	4.2–5.4 × 10¹²/L
Children (varies with age)	4.5–5.1 million/mm³	4.5–5.1 × 10¹²/L
Leukocytes		
Total	4500–11,000 mm³	4.5–11.0 × 10⁹/L

Differential	Percentage	Absolute	Absolute
Myelocytes	0	0/mm³	0/L
Band neutrophils	3–5	150–400/mm³	150–400 × 10⁶/L
Segmented neutrophils	54–62	3000–5800/mm³	3000–5800 × 10⁶/L
Lymphocytes	25–33	1500–3000/mm³	1500–3000 × 10⁶/L
Monocytes	3–7	300–500/mm³	300–500 × 10⁶/L
Eosinophils	1–3	50–250/mm³	50–250 × 10⁶/L
Basophils	0–1	15–50/mm³	15–50 × 10⁶/L

	Conventional Units	SI Units
Platelets	150,000–400,000/mm³	150–400 × 10⁹/L
Reticulocytes	25,000–75,000/mm³ (0.5–1.5% of erythrocytes)	25–75 × 10⁹/L
Coagulation tests		
Bleeding time (template)	2.75–8.0 min	2.75–8.0 min
Coagulation time (glass tubes)	5–15 min	5–15 min
D-Dimer	< 0.5 µg/mL	< 0.5 mg/L
Factor VIII and other coagulation factors	50–150% of normal	0.5–1.5 of normal
Fibrin split products (Thrombo–Welco test)	< 10 µg/mL	< 10 mg/L
Fibrinogen	200–400 mg/dL	2.0–4.0 g/L
Partial thromboplastin time (PTT)	20–35 sec	20–35 s
Prothrombin time (PT)	12.0–14.0 sec	12.0–14.0 s
Coombs' test		
Direct	Negative	Negative
Indirect	Negative	Negative
Corpuscular values of erythrocytes		
Mean corpuscular hemoglobin (MCH)	26–34 pg/cell	26–34 pg/cell

Continued

Reference Values in Hematology
(continued)

	Conventional Units	SI Units
Mean corpuscular volume (MCV)	80–96 μm^3	80–96 fL
Mean corpuscular hemoglobin concentration (MCHC)	32–36 g/dL	320–360 g/L
Erythrocyte sedimentation rate (ESR)		
Wintrobe		
Males	0–5 mm/h	0–5 mm/h
Females	0–15 mm/h	0–15 mm/h
Westergren		
Males	0–15 mm/h	0–15 mm/h
Females	0–20 mm/h	0–20 mm/h
	20–165 mg/dL	0.20–1.65 g/L
Haptoglobin	26–185 mg/dL	260–1850 mg/L
Hematocrit		
Males	40–54 mL/dL	0.40–0.54 volume fraction
Females	37–47 mL/dL	0.37–0.47 volume fraction
Newborns	49–54 mL/dL	0.49–0.54 volume fraction
Children (varies with age)	35–49 mL/dL	0.35–0.49 volume fraction
Hemoglobin		
Males	14.0–18.0 gm/dL	2.17–2.79 mmol/L
Females	12.0–16.0 gm/dL	1.86–2.48 mmol/L
Newborns	16.5–19.5 gm/dL	2.56–3.02 mmol/L
Children (varies with age)	11.2–16.5 gm/dL	1.74–2.56 mmol/L
Hemoglobin, fetal	<1.0% of total	<0.01 of total
Hemoglobin A$_{1C}$	3–5% of total	0.03–0.05 of total
Hemoglobin A$_2$	1.5–3.0% of total	0.015–0.03 of total
Hemoglobin, plasma	0–5.0 mg/dL	0–0.8 μmol/L
Methemoglobin	30–130 mg/dL	4.7–20 μmol/L

From: Miller/Keane: Encyclopedia & Dictionary of Medicine, Nursing, & Allied Health (6th ed.). Philadelphia: WB Saunders, p.1843. Reprinted with permission.

Reference Values for Clinical Chemistry (Blood, Serum, and Plasma)

(For some procedures, the reference values may vary depending on the method used)

	Conventional Units	SI Units
Aspartate aminotransferase (AST, SGOT), serum	1–36 U/L	1–36 U/L
Base excess, arterial blood, calculated	0 ± 2 mEq/L	0 ± 2 mmol/L
β-carotene, serum	60–260 µg/dL	1.1–8.6 µmol/L
Bicarbonate		
Venous plasma	23–29 mEq/L	23–29 mmol/L
Arterial blood	18–23 mEq/L	18–23 mmol/L
Bile acids, serum	0.3–3.0 mg/dL	3–30 mg/L
Bilirubin, serum		
Conjugated	0.1–0.4 mg/dL	1.7–6.8 µmol/L
Total	0.3–1.1 mg/dL	5.1–19 µmol/L
Calcium, serum	9.0–11.0 mg/dL	2.25–2.75 mmol/L
Calcium, ionized, serum	4.25–5.25 mg/dL	1.05–1.30 mmol/L
Carbon dioxide, total, serum or plasma	24–30 mEq/L	24–30 mmol/L
Carbon dioxide tension (Pco_2), blood	35–45 mm Hg	35–45 mm Hg
Ceruloplasmin, serum	23–44 mg/dL	230–440 mg/L
Chloride, serum or plasma	96–106 mEq/L	96–106 mmol/L
Cholesterol, serum or EDTA plasma		
Desirable range	<200 mg/dL	<5.18 mmol/L
LDL cholesterol	60–180 mg/dL	600–1800 mg/L
HDL cholesterol	30–80 mg/dL	300–800 mg/L
Copper	70–140 µg/dL	11–22 µmol/L
Corticotropin (ACTH), plasma, 8 AM	10–80 pg/mL	2–18 pmol/L
Cortisol, plasma		
8 AM	6–23 µg/dL	170–635 nmol/L
4 PM	3–15 µg/dL	82–413 nmol/L
10 PM	<50% of 8 AM value	<0.5 of 8 AM value
Creatine, serum		
Males	0.2–0.5 mg/dL	15–40 µmol/L
Females	0.3–0.9 mg/dL	25–70 µmol/L
Creatine kinase (CK), serum		
Males	55–170 U/L	55–170 U/L
Females	30–135 U/L	30–135 U/L
Creatine kinase MB isoenzyme, serum	0.0–4.7 ng/mL	0.0–4.7 µg/L
Creatinine, serum	0.6–1.2 mg/dL	50–110 µmol/L

Continued

Reference Values for Clinical Chemistry (Blood, Serum, and Plasma) *(continued)*

(For some procedures, the reference values may vary depending on the method used)

Lab Values

	Conventional Units	SI Units
Estradiol–17β, adult		
Males	10–65 pg/mL	35–240 pmol/L
Females		
Follicular phase	30–100 pg/mL	110–370 pmol/L
Ovulatory phase	200–400 pg/mL	730–1470 pmol/L
Luteal phase	50–140 pg/mL	180–510 pmol/L
Ferritin, serum	20–200 ng/mL	20–200 µg/L
Fibrinogen, plasma	200–400 mg/dL	2.0–4.0 g/L
Folate, serum	1.8–9.0 ng/mL	4.1–20.4 nmol/L
Erythrocytes	150–450 ng/mL	340–1020 nmol/L
Follicle–stimulating hormone (FSH), plasma		
Males	4–25 mU/mL	4–25 U/L
Females	4–30 mU/mL	4–30 U/L
Postmenopausal	40–250 mU/mL	40–250 U/L
γ-Glutamyltransferase (GGT), serum	5–40 U/L	5–40 U/L
Gastrin, fasting, serum	0–110 pg/mL	0–110 ng/L
Glucose, fasting, plasma or serum	70–115 mg/dL	3.9–6.4 mmol/L
Growth hormone (hGH), plasma, adult, fasting	0–6 ng/mL	0–6 µg/L
Haptoglobin, serum	20–165 mg/dL	0.20–1.65 g/L
Immunoglobulins, serum (see Reference Values for Immunologic Procedures)		
Insulin, fasting, plasma	5–25 µU/mL	36–179 pmol/L
Iron, serum	75–175 µg/dL	13–31 µmol/L
Iron binding capacity, serum		
Total	250–410 µg/dL	45–73 µmol/L
Saturation	20–55%	0.20–0.55
Lactate		
Venous whole blood	5.0–20.0 mg/dL	0.60–2.2 mmol/L
Arterial whole blood	5.0–15.0 mg/dL	0.6–1.7 mmol/L
Lactate dehydrogenase (LD), serum	110–220 U/L	110–220 U/L
Lipase, serum	10–140 U/L	10–140 U/L

Continued

Reference Values for Clinical Chemistry (Blood, Serum, and Plasma) *(continued)*

(For some procedures, the reference values may vary depending on the method used)

	Conventional Units	SI Units
Lutotropin (LH), serum		
Males	1–9 U/L	1–9 U/L
Females		
Follicular phase	2–10 U/L	2–10 U/L
Midcycle peak	15–65 U/L	15–65 U/L
Luteal phase	1–12 U/L	1–12 U/L
Postmenopausal	12–65 U/L	12–65 U/L
Magnesium, serum	1.8–3.0 mg/dL	0.75–1.25 mmol/L
Osmolality	286–295 mOsm/kg water	285–295 mmol/kg water
Oxygen, blood, arterial, room air		
Partial pressure (PaO_2)	80–100 mm Hg	80–100 mm Hg
Saturation (SaO_2)	95–98%	95–98%
pH, arterial blood	7.35–7.45	7.35–7.45
Phosphate, inorganic, serum		
Adult	3.0–4.5 mg/dL	1.0–1.5 mmol/L
Child	4.0–7.0 mg/dL	1.3–2.3 mmol/L
Potassium		
Serum	3.5–5.0 mEq/L	3.5–5.0 mmol/L
Plasma	3.5–4.5 mEq/L	3.5–4.5 mmol/L
Progesterone, serum, adult		
Males	0.0–0.4 ng/mL	0.0–1.3 mmol/L
Females		
Follicular phase	0.1–1.5 ng/mL	0.3–4.8 mmol/L
Luteal phase	2.5–28.0 ng/mL	8.0–89.0 mmol/L
Prolactin, serum		
Males	1.0–15.0 ng/mL	1.0–15.0 µg/L
Females	1.0–20.0 ng/mL	1.0–20.0 µg/L
Protein, serum, electrophoresis		
Total	6.0–8.0 g/dL	60–80 g/L
Albumin	3.5–5.5 g/dL	35–55 g/L
Alpha$_1$ globulin	0.2–0.4g/dL	2–4 g/L
Alpha$_2$ globulin	0.5–0.9 g/dL	5–9 g/L
Beta globulin	0.6–1.1 g/dL	6–11 g/L
Gamma globulin	0.7–1.7 g/dL	7–17 g/L
Pyruvate, blood	0.3–0.9 mg/dL	0.03–0.10 mmol/L
Rheumatoid factor	0.0–30.0 IU/mL	0.0–30.0 KIU/mL
Sodium, serum or plasma	135–145 mEq/L	135–145 mmol/L

Continued

Reference Values for Clinical Chemistry (Blood, Serum, and Plasma)
(continued)

(For some procedures, the reference values may vary depending on the method used)

	Conventional Units	SI Units
Testosterone, plasma		
Males, adult	300–1200 ng/dL	10.4–41.6 nmol/L
Females, adult	20–75 ng/dL	0.7–2.6 nmol/L
Pregnant females	40–200 ng/dL	1.4–6.9 nmol/L
Thyroglobulin	3–42 ng/mL	3–42 µg/L
Thyrotropin (hTSH), serum	0.4–4.8 µIU/mL	0.4–4.8 mIU/L
Thyrotropin–releasing hormone (TRH)	5–60 pg/mL	5–60 ng/L
Thyroxine, free (FT_4), serum	0.9–2.1 ng/dL	12–27 pmol/L
Thyroxine, (T_4), serum	4.5–12.0 µg/dL	58–154 nmol/L
Thyroxine–binding globulin (TBG)	15.0–34.0 µg/mL	15.0–34.0 mg/L
Transferrin	250–430 mg/dL	2.5–4.3 g/L
Triglycerides, serum, after 12-hr fast	40–150 mg/dL	0.4–1.5 g/L
Triiodothyronine (T_3), serum	70–190 ng/dL	1.1–2.9 nmol/L
Triiodothyronine uptake, resin (T_3RU)	25–38% uptake	0.25–0.38 uptake
Urate		
Males	2.5–8.0 mg/dL	150–480 µmol/L
Females	2.2–7.0 mg/dL	130–420 µmol/L
Urea, serum or plasma	24–49 mg/dL	4.0–8.2 nmol/L
Urea nitrogen, serum or plasma	11–23 mg/dL	8.0–16.4 nmol/L
Viscosity, serum	1.4–1.8 times water	1.4–1.8 times water
Vitamin A, serum	20–80 µg/dL	0.70–2.80 µmol/L
Vitamin B_{12}, serum	180–900 pg/mL	133–664 pmol/L

From: Miller/Keane: Encyclopedia & Dictionary of Medicine, Nursing, & Allied Health (6th ed.). Philadelphia: WB Saunders, p.1844-1845. Reprinted with permission.

Lab Values

Reference Values for Therapeutic Drug Monitoring

	Therapeutic Range	Toxic Levels	Proprietary Names
Analgesics			
Acetaminophen	10–20 µg/mL	>250 µg/mL	Tylenol, Datril
Salicylate	100–250 µg/mL	>300 µg/mL	Aspirin, Bufferin
Antibiotics			
Amikacin	25–30 µg/mL	Peak: >35 µg/mL	Amikin
		Trough: > 0 µg/mL	
Chloramphenicol	10–20 µg/mL	>25 µg/mL	Chloromycetin
Gentamicin	5–10 µg/mL	Peak: > 0 µg/mL	Garamycin
		Trough: >2 µg/mL	
Tobramycin	5–10 µg/mL	Peak: > 0 µg/mL	Nebcin
		Trough: >2 µg/mL	
Vancomycin	5–10 µg/mL	Peak: >40 µg/mL	Vancocin
		Trough: >10 µg/mL	
Anticonvulsants			
Carbamazepine	5–12 µg/mL	>15 µg/mL	Tegretol
Ethosuximide	40–100 µg/mL	>150 µg/mL	Zarontin

Continued

Lab Values

Reference Values for Therapeutic Drug Monitoring *(continued)*

	Therapeutic Range	Toxic Levels	Proprietary Names
Phenobarbital	15–40 µg/mL	40–100 ng/mL (varies widely)	Luminal
Phenytoin	10–20 µg/mL	>20 µg/mL	Dilantin
Primidone	5–12 µg/mL	>15 µg/mL	Mysoline
Valproic acid	50–100 µg/mL	>100 µg/mL	Depakene
Antineoplastics and Immunosuppressives			
Cyclosporine	50–400 ng/mL	>400 ng/mL	Sandimmune
Methotrexate, high dose, 48 hr	Variable	> 1 µmol/L 4 hr after dose	Mexate, Folex
Tacrolimus (FK–506), whole blood	3–10 µg/L	>15 µg/L	Prognaf
Bronchodilators and Respiratory Stimulants			
Caffeine	3–15 ng/mL	>30 ng/mL	
Theophylline (aminophylline)	10–20 µg/mL	>20 µg/mL	Elixophyllin, Quibron
Cardiovascular Drugs			
Amiodarone (specimen must be obtained more than 8 h after last dose)	1.0–2.0 µg/mL	2.0 µg/mL	Cordarone

Continued

Reference Values for Therapeutic Drug Monitoring *(continued)*

	Therapeutic Range	Toxic Levels	Proprietary Names
Digitoxin (specimen must be obtained 12–24 h after last dose)	15–25 ng/mL	>25 ng/mL	Crystodigin
Digoxin (specimen must be obtained more than 6 h after last dose)	0.8–2.0 ng/mL	>2.4 ng/mL	Lanoxin
Disopyramide	2–5 µg/mL	>5 µg/mL	Norpace
Flecainide	0.2–1.0 ng/mL	>1 ng/mL	Tambocor
Lidocaine	1.5–5.0 µg/mL	>6–8 µg/mL	Xylocaine
Procainamide	4–10 µg/mL	>12 µg/mL	Pronestyl
Procainamide plus NAPA	8–30 µg/mL	>30 µg/mL	
Propranolol	50–100 ng/mL	Variable	Inderal
Quinidine	2–5 µg/mL	>10 µg/mL	Quinaglute
Tocainide	4–10 ng/mL	>10 ng/mL	Tonocard
Psychopharmacologic Drugs			
Amitriptyline	120–150 ng/mL	>500 ng/mL	Elavil
Bupropion	25–100 ng/mL	Not applicable	Triavil, Wellbutrin

Continued

Reference Values for Therapeutic Drug Monitoring *(continued)*

	Therapeutic Range	Toxic Levels	Proprietary Names
Desipramine	150–300 ng/mL	>500 ng/mL	Norpramin, Pertofrane
Imipramine	125–250 ng/mL	>400 ng/mL	Tofranil
Lithium (obtain specimen 12 h after last dose)	0.6–1.5 mEq/L	>1.5 mEq/L	Lithobid, Janimine
Nortriptyline	50–150 ng/mL	>500 ng/mL	Aventyl, Pamelor

From: Miller/Keane: Encyclopedia & Dictionary of Medicine, Nursing, & Allied Health (6th ed.). Philadelphia: WB Saunders, p.1846. Reprinted with permission.

Reference Values for Clinical Chemistry (Urine)

(For some procedures, the reference values may vary depending on the method used)

	Conventional Units	SI Units
Acetone and acetoacetate, qualitative	Negative	Negative
Albumin		
Qualitative	Negative	Negative
Quantitative	10–100 mg/24 hr	0.15–1.5 µmol/day
Aldosterone	3–20 µg/24 hr	8.3–55 nmol/day
δ-Aminolevulinic acid (δ-ALA)	1.3–7.0 mg/24 hr	10–53 µmol/day
Amylase	<17 U/hr	<17 U/hr
Amylase/creatinine clearance ratio	0.01–0.04	0.01–0.04
Bilirubin, qualitative	Negative	Negative
Calcium (regular diet)	<250 mg/24 hr	<6.3 mmol/day
Catecholamines		
Epinephrine	<10 µg/24 hr	<55 nmol/day
Norepinephrine	<100 µg/24 hr	<590 nmol/day
Total free catecholamines	4–126 µg/24 hr	24–745 nmol/day
Total metanephrines	0.1–1.6 mg/24 hr	0.5–8.1 µmol/day
Chloride (varies with intake)	110–250 mEq/24 hr	110–250 mmol/day
Copper	0–50 µg/24 hr	0–0.80 µmol/day
Cortisol, free	10–100 µg/24 hr	27.6–276 nmol/day
Creatine		
Males	0–40 mg/24 hr	0.0–0.30 mmol/day
Females	0–80 mg/24 hr	0.0–0.60 mmol/day
Creatinine	15–25 mg/kg/24 hr	0.13–0.22 mmol/kg/day
Creatinine clearance (endogenous)		
Males	110–150 mL/min/1.73 m^2	110–150 mL/min/1.73 m^2
Females	105–132 mL/min/1.73 m^2	105–132 mL/min/1.73 m^2
Cystine or cysteine	Negative	Negative
Dehydroepiandrosterone		
Males	0.2–2.0 mg/24 hr	0.7–6.9 µmol/day
Females	0.2–1.8 mg/24 hr	0.7–6.2 µmol/day
Estrogens, total		
Males	4–25 µg/24 hr	14–90 nmol/day
Females	5–100 µg/24 hr	18–360 nmol/day
Glucose (as reducing substance)	<250 mg/24 hr	<250 mg/day
Hemoglobin and myoglobin, qualitative	Negative	Negative
Homogentisic acid, qualitative	Negative	Negative

Continued

Reference Values for Clinical Chemistry (Urine) *(continued)*

	Conventional Units	SI Units
17–Hydroxycorticosteroids		
Males	3–9 mg/24 hr	8.3–25 µmol/day
Females	2–8 mg/24 hr	5.5–22 µmol/day
5–Hydroxyindoleacetic acid		
Qualitative	Negative	Negative
Quantitative	2–6 mg/24 hr	10–31 µmol/day
17–Ketogenic steroids		
Males	5–23 mg/24 hr	17–80 µmol/day
Females	3–15 mg/24 hr	10–52 µmol/day
17–Ketosteroids		
Males	8–22 mg/24 hr	28–76 µmol/day
Females	6–15 mg/24 hr	21–52 µmol/day
Magnesium	6–10 mEq/24 hr	3–5 mmol/day
Metanephrines	0.05–1.2 ng/mg creatinine	0.30–0.70 mmol/ mmol creatinine
Osmolality	38–1400 mOsm/ kg water	38–1400 mOsm/ kg water
pH	4.6–8.0	4.6–8.0
Phenylpyruvic acid, qualitative	Negative	Negative
Phosphate	0.4–1.3 grams/24 hr	13–42 mmol/day
Porphobilinogen		
Qualitative	Negative	Negative
Quantitative	< 2.0 mg/24 hr	< 9 µmol/day
Porphyrins		
Coproporphyrin	50–250 µg/24 hr	77–380 nmol/day
Uroporphyrin	10–30 µg/24 hr	12–36 nmol/day
Potassium	25–125 mEq/24 hr	25–125 mmol/day
Pregnanediol		
Males	0.0–1.9 mg/24 hr	0.0–6.0 µmol/day
Females		
Proliferativephase	0.0–2.6 mg/24 hr	0.0–8.0 µmol/day
Luteal phase	2.6–10.6 mg/24 hr	8–33 µmol/day
Postmenopausal	0.2–1.0 mg/24 hr	0.6–3.1 µmol/day
Pregnanetriol	0.0–2.5 mg/24 hr	0.0–7.4 µmol/day
Protein, total		
Qualitative	Negative	Negative
Quantitative	10–150 mg/24 hr	10–150 mg/day
Protein/creatinine ratio	<0.2	<0.2
Sodium (regular diet)	60–260 mEq/24 hr	60–260 mmol/day
Specific gravity	1.003–1.030	1.003–1.030
Random specimen	1.003–1.030	1.003–1.030
24–hour collection	1.015–1.025	1.015–1.025
Urate (regular diet)	250–750 mg/24 hr	1.5–4.4 mmol/day
Urobilinogen	0.5–4.0 mg/24 hr	0.6–6.8 µmol/day
Vanillylmandelic acid (VMA)	1–8 mg/24 hr	5–40 µmol/24 h

From: Miller/Keane: Encyclopedia & Dictionary of Medicine, Nursing, & Allied Health (6th ed.). Philadelphia: WB Saunders, p.1847-1848. Reprinted with permission.

Common Causes of Variations in the Appearance of Urine

Colorless	Dilute urine as seen in high fluid intake, diabetes insipidus, diuretic therapy, diabetes mellitus
Cloudy	Phosphate precipitation (normal in aging urine specimens), pyuria; bacteriuria, epithelial cells, blood, leukocytes
Smoky or hazy	Hemoglobin and remnants of red blood cells, chyle, prostatic fluid; yeast
Dark yellow or yellow-orange	Concentrated urine as seen in dehydration, low fluid intake, inability of the kidneys to dilute urine, bile
Yellow-brown	Bile
Orange-red	Pyridium, bile
Red or red-brown	Blood, ingestion of beets, berries, fava beans, excessive red food coloring, pyrvinium pamoate (Povan)
Green	Pseudomonas bacteria, bile pigments
Dark brown or black	Methylene blue, typhus

From: Miller/Keane: Encyclopedia & Dictionary of Medicine, Nursing, & Allied Health (6th ed.). Philadelphia: WB Saunders, p.1690. Reprinted with permission.

Lab Values

Lab Values

SI Units

Quantity	Unit	Symbol	Pronunciation	Derivation
Base Units				
length	meter	m	me′ter	
mass	kilogram	kg	kil′o-gram	
time	second	s	sek′und	
electric current	ampere	A	am′pēr	
temperature	kelvin	K	kel′vin	
luminous intensity	candela	cd	kan-del′ah	
amount of substance	mole	mol	mōl	
Supplementary Units				
plane angle	radian	rad	ra′de-an	
solid angle	steradian	sr	ste-ra′de-an	
Derived Units				
force	newton	N	noo′ton	$kg \cdot m/s^2$
pressure	pascal	Pa	pas′kal	N/m^2
energy, work	joule	J	jōōl	$N \cdot m$
power	watt	W	waht	J/s
electric charge	coulomb	C	koo′lom	$A \cdot s$
electric potential	volt	V	volt	J/C

Lab Values

electric capacitance	farad	F	far'ad	C/V
electric resistance	ohm	Ω	ōm	V/A
electric conductance	siemens	S	se'menz	$Ω^{-1}$
magnetic flux	weber	Wb	web'er	$V \cdot s$
magnetic flux density	tesla	T	tes'lah	Wb/m^2
inductance	henry	H	hen're	Wb/A
frequency	hertz	Hz	herts	s^{-1}
luminous flux	lumen	lm	loo'men	$cd \cdot sr$
illumination	lux	lx	luks	lm/m^2
temperature	degree celsius	°C	sel'se-us	$K-273.15$
radioactivity	becquerel	Bq	bek-er-el'	s^{-1}
absorbed dose	gray	Gy	gra	J/kg
absorbed dose equivalent	sievert	Sv	se'vert	J/kg

From: Miller/Keane: Encyclopedia & Dictionary of Medicine, Nursing, & Allied Health (6th ed.). Philadelphia: WB Saunders, p.1488. Reprinted with permission.

Prefixes for SI Units

Multiplication	Prefix	Symbol	Pronun-ciation
1 000 000 000 000 000 000 = 10^{18}	exa	E	ek'sah
1 000 000 000 000 000 = 10^{15}	peta	P	pet'ah
1 000 000 000 000 = 10^{12}	tera	T	ter'ah
1 000 000 000 = 10^{9}	giga	G	jig'ah
1 000 000 = 10^{6}	mega	M	meg'ah
1 000 = 10^{3}	kilo	k	kil'o
1 00 = 10^{2}	hecto	h	hek'to
10 = 10	deka	dk	dek'ah
0.1 = 10^{-1}	deci	d	des'ī
0.01 = 10^{-2}	centi	c	sen'tī
0.001 = 10^{-3}	milli	m	mil'ī
0.000001 = 10^{-6}	micro	μ	mi'kro
0.000 000 001 = 10^{-9}	nano	n	nan'o
0.000 000 000 001 = 10^{-12}	pico	p	pi'ko
0.000 000 000 000 001 = 10^{-15}	femto	f	fem'to
0.000 000 000 000 000 001 = 10^{-18}	atto	a	at'o

From: Miller/Keane: Encyclopedia & Dictionary of Medicine, Nursing, & Allied Health (6th ed.). Philadelphia: WB Saunders, p.1489. Reprinted with permission.

Lab Values

Medical Language

Selected Word Parts

Suffixes that pertain to symptoms and diagnosis

-algia,-dynia	pain
-cele	hernia
-ectasis	dilation, stretching
-edema	swelling
-emesis	vomiting
-ia, -iasis	condition
-itis	inflammation
-lepsy	seizure
-malacia	abnormal softness
-mania	excessive preoccupation
-oid	resembling
-oma	tumor
-osis	condition, disease
-pathy	disease
-ptosis	prolapse, sagging
-rrhexis	rupture
-rrhagia	hemorrhage
-rrhea	flow, discharge
-sclerosis	hardening
-stasis	stopping, controlling

Suffixes that pertain to surgery

-centesis	puncture
-ectomy	excision, surgical removal
-lysis	destruction
-pexy	surgical fixation
-plasty	repair
-rrhaphy	suture
-scope	instrument used for viewing
-scopy	visually examining
-stomy	forming artificial opening
-tome	cutting instrument
-tomy	incision
-tripsy	crushing

Continued

Selected Word Parts *(continued)*

Combining forms that denote color

alb/o, albin/o	white
chlor/o	green
chrom/o	color
cyan/o	blue
erythr/o	red
leuc/o, leuk/o	white
melan/o	black
xanth/o	yellow

Word parts that describe number or quantity

a-, an-	without, no, absent
bi-	two
di-	two, twice
diplo-	double
hemi, semi-	half
hyper-	greater than normal, excessive
hypo-	less than normal
mono-, uni-	one
multi-, poly-	many
nulli-	none
-penia	deficiency
primi-	first
quadri-	four
tetra-	four
tri-	three

Word parts that pertain to size

macr/o, megal/o	large
micr/o, -ole	small

Word parts that pertain to body fluids

chol/e	bile
dacry/o	tear
-emia, hem/a, hem/o, hemat/o	blood

Continued

Selected Word Parts *(continued)*

hidr/o	sweat
hydr/o	water
lymph/o	lymph
muc/o, myx/o	mucus
py/o	pus
sial/o	saliva
ur/o	urine

Combining forms that pertain to body substances

lip/o	fat
calc/i	calcium
glyc/o	sugar
lith/o	stone, calculus
thromb/o	clot

From: Leonard, P. (2000). Quick and Easy Medical Terminology (3rd ed.). Philadelphia: WB Saunders, Inside Cover (Selected Word Parts). Reprinted with Permission.

Medical Language

Medical Terminology → English

Word Part	*Meaning*
a-, an-	no, not
ab-	away from
abdomin/o	abdomen
-ac	pertaining to
ad-	toward
aden/o	gland
adren/o	adrenal gland
-al	pertaining to
-algia	pain
alveol/o	alveolus (air sac within the lung)
amni/o	amnion (sac that surrounds the embryo)
-an	pertaining to
ana-	up, apart
an/o	anus
angi/o	vessel (blood)
ante-	before, forward
anti-	against
append/o, appendic/o	appendix
-ar	pertaining to
arteri/o	artery
arteriol/o	small artery
arthr/o	joint
-ary	pertaining to
-ation	process, condition
axill/o	armpit
balan/o	penis
bi-	two
bi/o	life
brady-	slow
bronch/o	bronchial tube
bronchiol/o	small bronchial tube
calcane/o	calcaneus (heel bone)
capillar/o	capillary
carcin/o	cancer, cancerous
cardi/o	heart
carp/o	wrist bones (carpals)
-cele	hernia
-centesis	surgical puncture to remove fluid
cephal/o	head
cerebell/o	cerebellum (posterior part of the brain)
cerebr/o	cerebrum (largest part of the brain)
cervic/o	neck
chem/o	drug, chemical
cholecyst/o	gallbladder
choledoch/o	common bile duct
chondr/o	cartilage
chron/o	time

Continued

Medical Language

Word Part	Meaning
-cision	process of cutting
cis/o	to cut
clavicul/o	clavicle (collar bone)
-coccus	berry-shaped bacteria (pl. cocci)
coccyg/o	tailbone
col/o	colon (large intestine)
colon/o	colon
colp/o	vagina
comi/o	to care for
con-	with, together
coni/o	dust
-coniosis	abnormal condition of dust
coron/o	heart
cost/o	rib
crani/o	skull
crin/o	secrete
-crine	secretion
-crit	separate
cry/o	cold
cutane/o	skin
cyst/o	urinary bladder
cyt/o	cell
-cyte	cell
dermat/o, derm/o	skin
dia-	through, complete
dur/o	dura mater (outermost meningeal layer)
dys-	painful, abnormal, bad, difficult
-eal	pertaining to
ec-	out, outside
ecto-	out, outside
-ectomy	excision (resection, removal)
-emesis	vomiting
-emia	blood condition
en-	within, in, inner
encephal/o	brain
endo-	within, in, inner
endocrin/o	endocrine glands
endometri/o	endometrium (inner lining of the uterus)
enter/o	intestines (usually small intestine)
epi-	above, upon
epiglott/o	epiglottis
epitheli/o	skin (surface tissue)
erythr/o	red
esophag/o	esophagus
esthesi/o	sensation
ex-, extra-	out, outside
femor/o	femur, thigh bone
fibul/o	fibula (smaller lower leg bone)
gastr/o	stomach
gen/o	to produce

Continued

Medical Language

Word Part	Meaning
-gen	to produce
-genesis	producing, forming
-genic	pertaining to producing, produced by
ger/o	old age
glyc/o	sugar
gnos/o	knowledge
-gram	record
-graphy	process of recording, to record
gynec/o	woman, female
hemat/o, hem/o	blood
hepat/o	liver
humer/o	humerus (upper arm bone)
hyper-	excessive, above
hypo-	below, deficient
hypophys/o	pituitary gland
hyster/o	uterus
-ia	condition
iatr/o	treatment
-ic	pertaining to
ile/o	ileum (third part of small intestine)
ili/o	ilium (upper part of hip bone)
in-	in, into
-ine	pertaining to
inguin/o	groin
inter-	between
intra-	within
-ior	pertaining to
isch/o	to hold back
-ism	condition, process
-ist	specialist
-itis	inflammation
lapar/o	abdomen
laryng/o	larynx (voice box)
later/o	side
leuk/o	white
-listhesis	to slip, slide
lith/o	stone
-lith	stone
-logy	study of
lumb/o	loin, waist region
lymph/o	lymph
lymphaden/o	lymph nodes
lymphangi/o	lymph vessel
lys/o	separation, breakdown, destruction
-lysis	separation, breakdown, destruction
mal-	bad
mamm/o	breast
mast/o	breast
mediastin/o	mediastinum
medull/o	medulla oblongata (lower part of the brain)

Continued

Word Part	**Meaning**
-megaly	enlargement
men/o	menstruation
mening/o	meninges (membranes covering brain and spinal cord)
meta-	beyond, change
metacarp/o	metacarpals (hand bones)
metatars/o	metatarsals (foot bones)
metr/o	uterus; to measure
-metry	measurement
-mortem	death
-motor	movement
muscul/o	muscle
my/o	muscle
myel/o	bone marrow (with -blast, -oma, -cyte, -genic)
myel/o	spinal cord (with -gram, -itis, -cele)
myos/o	muscle
myring/o	eardrum
nas/o	nose
nat/i	birth
neo-	new
nephr/o	kidney
neur/o	nerve
nos/o	disease
obstetr/o	midwife
ocul/o	eye
-oma	tumor, mass, swelling
onc/o	tumor
oophor/o	ovary
ophthalm/o	eye
-opsy	process of viewing
opt/o	eye
or/o	mouth
orch/o	testicle, testis
orchi/o	testicle, testis
orchid/o	testicle, testis
orth/o	straight
-osis	abnormal condition
oste/o	bone
ot/o	ear
-ous	pertaining to
ovari/o	ovary
pancreat/o	pancreas
para-	beside, near, along the side of
-partum	birth
path/o	disease
-pathy	disease condition
ped/o	child
pelv/o	hip bone
per-	through
peri-	surrounding

Continued

Medical Language

Word Part	Meaning
peritone/o	peritoneum (membrane around abdominal organs)
perone/o	fibula
-pexy	fixation (surgical)
phalang/o	phalanges (finger and toe bones)
pharyng/o	pharynx, throat
-philia	attraction to
phleb/o	vein
phren/o	diaphragm
phren/o	mind
plas/o	formation, growth, development
-plasm	formation, growth, development
-plasty	surgical repair
-plegia	paralysis
pleur/o	pleura (membranes surrounding the lungs)
-pnea	breathing
pneum/o	air, lung
pneumon/o	lung
-poiesis	formation
post-	after, behind
pre-	before
pro-, pros-	before, forward
proct/o	anus and rectum
prostat/o	prostate gland
psych/o	mind
-ptosis	prolapse, sagging
-ptysis	spitting
pulmon/o	lung
pyel/o	renal pelvis (central section of the kidney)
radi/o	x-ray; radius (lateral lower arm bone)
re-, retro-	behind, back
rect/o	rectum
ren/o	kidney
retin/o	retina of the eye
rheumat/o	flow, fluid
rhin/o	nose
-rrhage	bursting forth of blood
-rrhagia	bursting forth of blood
-rrhea	flow, discharge
sacr/o	sacrum
salping/o	fallopian (uterine) tube; eustachian tube
-salpinx	fallopian (uterine) tube; eustachian tube
sarc/o	flesh
scapul/o	shoulder blade (bone)
-sclerosis	condition of hardening
-scope	instrument to view or visually examine
-scopy	process of viewing or visual examination
scrot/o	scrotal sac, scrotum
-section	to cut
-sept/o	infection
septic/o	infection
-sis	condition

Continued

Word Part	**Meaning**
-somatic	pertaining to the body
son/o	sound
-spasm	constriction
spin/o	backbone
splen/o	spleen
spondyl/o	vertebra, backbone
-stasis	stop, control; place, to stand
-stat	stop, control
stern/o	sternum (breast bone)
-stomy	opening
sub-	under, below
sym-	with, together (use before b, p, and m)
syn-	with, together
tachy-	fast
-tension	pressure
theli/o	nipple
-therapy	treatment
-thesis	to put or place
thorac/o	chest
thromb/o	clot
thymlo	thymus gland
thyr/o, thyroid/o	thyroid gland
tib/o	tibia or shin bone (larger lower leg bone)
-tic	pertaining to
-tomy	incision, process of cutting
tonsill/o	tonsils
top/o	to put, place
trache/o	trachea (windpipe)
trans-	across, through
tri-	three
troph/o	development, nourishment
-trophy	development, nourishment
tympan/o	eardrum
uln/o	ulna (medial lower arm bone)
ultra-	beyond
-um	structure
uni-	one
ureter/o	ureter
urethr/o	urethra
ur/o	urine, urinary tract
-uria	urine condition
uter/o	uterus
vagin/o	vagina
vas/o	vessel, vas deferens
vascul/o	blood vessel
ven/o	vein
vertebr/o	vertebra (backbone)
vesic/o	urinary bladder
-y	condition; process

Medical Language

From: Chabner, D. (1999). *Medical Terminology: A Short Course* (2nd edition).
Philadelphia: WB Saunders, p. 273-282. Reprinted with permission.

Spelling Prescriptions

Rules	Examples	Exceptions
I before E except after C and when the word sounds like AY, as in SAY	relieve receive neighbor weigh	either foreign height seizure
Drop final silent E when adding a suffix that begins with a vowel	achieve–achieving care–caring	change–changeable
Keep final silent E when adding a suffix that begins with a consonant	achieve–achievement care–careful	argue–argument judge–judgment true–truly
When adding -ING to a word that ends in IE, replace the IE with Y	die–dying tie–tying	
Double the final consonant of a one-syllable word when adding a suffix that begins with a vowel unless there are two vowels or another consonant before the final consonant	trim–trimming look–looking test–testing	

Plurals

Add S to most words	disease–diseases wound–wounds
Words that end in a consonant + Y: change the Y to an I and add ES	laboratory–laboratories pregnancy–pregnancies
Words that end in S, SH, CH, and X: add ES	crutch–crutches
Words that end in SIS: change to SES	diagnosis–diagnoses urinalysis–urinalyses
Words that end in a vowel + O: add S	radio–radios
Words that end in a consonant + O: add ES	echo–echoes

From: Haroun, L. (2000). Career Development for Health Professionals. Phila.: W B Saunders, p. 114, Table 5-4. Reprinted with permission.

Medical Language

Commonly Misspelled Words

absence	criticize	impatient
absorption	decision	indefinitely
accessible	definitely	infinite
accidentally	describe	intelligence
accommodate	despair	interesting
accumulate	develop	jewelry
achievement	discipline	judgment
acknowledge	disease	knowledge
acquire	efficiency	knowledgeable
address	eighth	label
affiliated	eligible	laboratory
aggravate	eliminate	legitimate
analyze	embarrass	leisure
appropriate	emphasize	license
assistant	encourage	loneliness
association	enthusiastic	magazine
athlete	entirely	maintenance
beginning	environment	management
behavior	equipped	maneuver
belief	equivalent	marriage
beneficial	especially	miscellaneous
bureau	exaggerate	necessary
business	exercise	negligible
businesses	exhausted	negligence
cafeteria	experience	neighbor
caffeine	extremely	noticeable
calendar	fascinate	obstacle
cancel	fatigue	occasion
canceled	February	occasionally
column	fluctuation	occur
coming	foreign	occurrence
committee	forty	often
commitment	fourth	original
committed	fragile	pamphlet
communicate	friend	parallel
comparative	government	particular
competition	harass	patience
cooperate	harassment	perform
correspond	height	persistent
criticism	hygiene	physically

Continued

Medical Language

physician	sensible
pneumonia	separate
possession	several
practical	severely
precede	significance
preference	similar
prejudice	sincerely
privilege	strategy
probably	strictly
proceed	substantial
prominent	succeed
psychiatry	success
psychology	surprise
qualified	sympathy
quantity	technique
questionnaire	temperature
quiet	thorough
quite	though
receipt	tongue
receive	transferred
recognize	typical
recommend	until
reference	urgent
resuscitate	useful
rhythm	usually
safety	vacuum
satisfactory	vague
schedule	vegetable
scissors	view
secretary	Wednesday
seize	weight
seizure	writing

From: Haroun, L. (2000). Career Development for Health Professionals. Phila.: W B Saunders, p. 115, Table 5-5. Reprinted with permission.

Commonly Confused Words

Word	Meaning	Sample Hints for Learning
accept	to take or receive	t<u>a</u>ke—<u>a</u>ccept
except	excluding, all but	<u>e</u>xclude—<u>e</u>xcept
access	way of entering	
excess	too much	e<u>x</u>tra—e<u>x</u>cess
adapt	adjust	adjust—ad<u>a</u>pt
adopt	to take as one's own	<u>o</u>wn—ad<u>o</u>pt
advice	helpful suggestions	
advise	to give advice	
affect	to influence	
effect	result; to bring about	
allowed	permitted	
aloud	capable of being heard	<u>loud</u> sound
already	before now, so soon	
all ready	completely prepared	It's <u>all</u> done.
capital	offficial seat of government; form of wealth	
capitol	building in which members of government meet	
choose	to select	
chose	selected (past tense of "choose")	
coarse	rough	The dog has a rough <u>coat</u>.
course	class; path or track	<u>Our</u> class is on track.
conscience	part of the mind that determines right and wrong	
conscious	awake; aware	
council	governing body	
counsel	advice; to give advice	
defer	delay	
differ	to be different; to disagree	<u>differ</u>—<u>differ</u>ent
desert	dry land area	1 rain <u>s</u>hower in the desert.
dessert	eaten at the end of a meal	2 cups of <u>s</u>ugar in dessert
it's	contraction of "it is"	The apostrophe replaces a word
its	possessive form of "it"	
later	after the usual time	
latter	the second of two	2 Ts = 2nd of 2
lay	put or place something (past = laid)	
lie	rest on a surface (past = lay!! - confusing!!)	
lead	type of metal; to guide; connecting wire	
led	guided (past tense of "lead")	

Continued

Medical Language

Commonly Confused Words *(continued)*

Word	Meaning	Sample Hints for Learning
loose	not tight	Bigger word, like a shirt, is looser
lose	to be unable to find	I lost one O.
maybe	perhaps	
may be	possible, permissible	
miner	mine worker	
minor	younger than the legal age	
overdo	to do too much	
overdue	late or past due	
patience	quality of being uncomplaining, unhurried	
patients	people under medical care	
passed	went by, earned a satisfactory grade	
past	before now, ended	
personal	private	
personnel	employees	
principal	head of a school, main or most important	The princi<u>pal</u> is your <u>pal</u>.
principle	general truth or rule	
stationary	not moving	S<u>t</u>ay in one place
stationery	paper for writing letters	L<u>e</u>tters are written on stationery
than	compared to	
then	at that time	
their	possessive of they	
there	in that place	
they're	contraction of "they are"	Apostrophe stands for "a"
to	toward, for the purpose of	
too	also, very, more than enough	
two	2	
weather	climate conditions	Weather can be <u>wet</u> <u>and</u> windy
whether	introduces alternatives	
who's	contraction of "who is"	Apostrophe stands for "is"
whose	possessive of "who"	
you're	contraction of "you are"	Apostrophe stands for "a"
your	possessive of you	<u>Our</u> is possessive; so is <u>your</u>

From: Haroun, L. (2000). Career Development for Health Professionals. Phila.: W B Saunders, p. 116-117, Table 5-6. Reprinted with permission.

Medical Language

Patient Care Reference

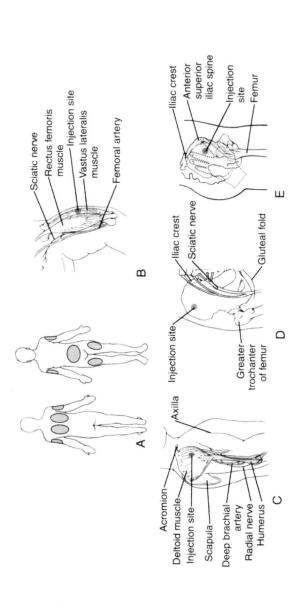

Sites for injections. A, subcutaneous injection sites. B, intramuscular injection site for children in the vastus lateralis muscle. C, D, and E, intramuscular injection sites for adults: C, deltoid muscle injection site. D, injection site in the buttock (dorsogluteal site). E, injection site in the anterolateral thigh (ventrogluteal site).

From: Miller/Keane: Encyclopedia & Dictionary of Medicine, Nursing, & Allied Health (6th ed.). Philadelphia: WB Saunders, p.832. Reprinted with permission.

Patient Care

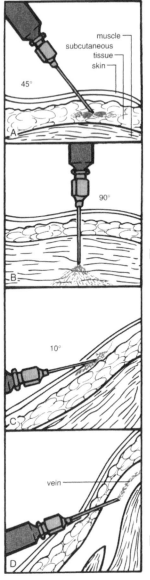

Subcutaneous

Intramuscular

Intradermal

Intravenous

Needle Insertion for Types of Injections

From: Leonard, P. (2001) IM to acc. Building a Medical Vocabulary (5th ed.). St. Louis: WB Saunders, TM 49 (Fig. 12-13 of text, p. 457). Reprinted with permission.

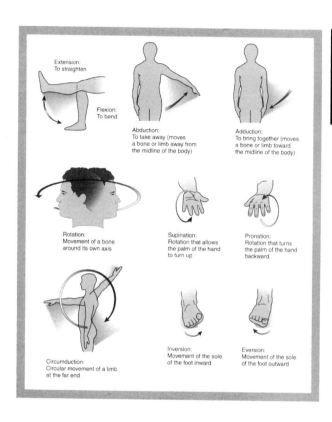

Types of Body Movements

From: Leonard, P. (2001) IM to acc. Building a Medical Vocabulary (5th ed.). St. Louis: WB Saunders, TM 40 (Fig. 10-16 of text, p. 366). Reprinted with permission.

TNM Staging System

T: Primary Tumor

TX	Primary tumor is not assessable
T0	No evidence of primary tumor
Tis	Carcinoma in situ
T1, T2, T3, T4	Progressive increase in tumor size and involvement locally

N: Regional Lymph Nodes

NX	Nodes are not assessable
N0	No metastasis to regional lymph nodes
N1, N2, N3	Increasing degrees of involvement of regional lymph nodes

Note: Extension of primary tumor directly into lymph nodes is considered metastasis to lymph nodes. Metastasis to a lymph node beyond the regional ones is considered to be a distant metastasis.

M: Distant Metastasis

MX	Presence of distant metastasis is not assessable
M0	No distant metastasis
MI	Presence of distant metastasis

From: Miller/Keane: Encyclopedia & Dictionary of Medicine, Nursing, & Allied Health (6th ed.). Philadelphia: WB Saunders, p.259. Reprinted with permission.

Burn Depth Categories

Degree	Cause	Surface Appearance	Color	Pain Level	Depth	Healing Time
First: minor except under the age of 18 months, over the age of 65 years, or if there is severe fluid loss	Flash flame, sunburn (ultraviolet)	Dry, no blisters, little or no edema	Erythematous	Painful	Epidermis only	2–5 days with no peeling or scarring; discoloration possible
Second: (partial thickness): Minor: adults, less than 15%, children less than 10% Moderate: adult 15%–30%, minor electrical or chemical. less than 15% but involving hands, feet, face, perineum, children: 10%–30% Severe: over 30%	Hot liquids or solids, flash flame, direct flame, chemical	Moist blebs and blisters	Mottled white to pink, red	Very painful	Epidermis; papillary and reticular layers of dermis, possibly fat domes of subcutaneous layer	Superficial: 5–21 days without grafting; deep 21–35; with infection, becomes full thickness
Third: (full thickness): Minor: less than 2% Moderate: 2%–10% or any involvement of hands, feet, face, perineum Severe: over 10% major chemical or electrical	Hot liquids or solids, flame, chemical, electrical	Dry leathery eschar; charred vessels visible under eschar	Mixed white waxy, pearly; dark khaki, mahogany; charred	Little or no pain	Subcutaneous tissue, may include fascia, muscle, and bone	Smaller areas may heal from edges in several weeks large areas require grafting, may take many months

From: Miller/Keane: Encyclopedia & Dictionary of Medicine, Nursing, & Allied Health (6th ed.), Philadelphia: WB Saunders, p.246. Reprinted with permission.

Patient Care

Apgar Scoring Chart

Sign	*0*	*1*	*2*
Heart rate	Absent	Below 100	Over 100
Respiratory effort	Absent	Slow, irregular	Good, crying
Muscle tone	Limp	Some flexion of extremities	Active motion
Response to catheter in nostril (tested after oro-pharynx is clear)	No response	Grimace	Cough or sneeze
Color	Blue, pale	Body pink, extremities blue	Completely pink

From: Miller/Keane: Encyclopedia & Dictionary of Medicine, Nursing, & Allied Health (6th ed.). Philadelphia: WB Saunders, p.116. Reprinted with permission.

Patient Care

Symbols & Time

Symbols Commonly Used in Clinical Practice

Symbols & Time

a	before
p̄	after
c̄	with
s̄	without
=	equal
≠	unequal
>	greater than
<	less than
↑	increase
↗	increasing
↓	decrease
↘	decreasing
−	negative, minus, deficiency, alkaline reaction
±	very slight trace or reaction, indefinite
+	slight trace or reaction, positive, plus, excess, acid reaction
+ +	trace or notable reaction
+ + +	moderate amount or reaction
+ + + +	large amount or pronounced reaction
#	number, pound, has been given or done
→	yields, leads to
←	resulting from or secondary to
(catalyst) ⟶	accelerant, increases velocity of a chemical reaction or process
♂ ○ ○ or □	male
♀ or ○	female
ʒ	dram
℥	ounce
1°, 2°	primary, secondary

From: Miller/Keane: Encyclopedia & Dictionary of Medicine, Nursing, & Allied Health (6th ed.). Philadelphia: WB Saunders, p.1802. Reprinted with permission.

Symbols & Time

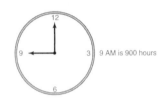

9 AM is 900 hours

From noon to midnight, 12 is added to the PM time.

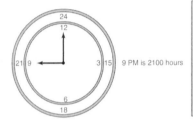

9 PM is 2100 hours

Noon is 1200 hours
1 PM is 1300 hours
2 PM is 1400 hours
3 PM is 1500 hours
4 PM is 1600 hours
5 PM is 1700 hours
6 PM is 1800 hours
7 PM is 1900 hours
8 PM is 2000 hours
9 PM is 2100 hours
10 PM is 2200 hours
11 PM is 2300 hours
Midnight is 2400 hours

Twenty-Four Hour Clock

The 24-hour clock (also known as military time) is used to standardize time and avoid the misinterpretation of charting entries related to AM and PM.

From midnight to noon, there is no difference between a 24-hour clock and the time as it is normally noted.

From: Miller/Keane: Encyclopedia & Dictionary of Medicine, Nursing, & Allied Health (6th ed.). Philadelphia: WB Saunders, p.1801. Reprinted with permission.

Tables of Weights and Measures

Metric—Apothecaries' Liquid Measure

Milliliters	Minims	Milliliters	Fluid Drams	Milliliters	Fluid Ounces
1	16.231	5	1.35	30	1.01
2	32.5	10	2.71	40	1.35
3	48.7	15	4.06	50	1.69
4	64.9	20	5.4	500	16.91
5	81.1	25	6.76	1000 (1 L)	33.815
		30	7.1		

Apothecaries'—Metric Liquid Measure

Minims	Milliliters	Minims	Milliliters
1	0.06	**Fluid Ounces**	
2	0.12	1	29.57
3	0.19	2	59.15
4	0.25	3	88.72
5	0.31	4	118.29
10	0.62	5	147.87
15	0.92	6	177.44
20	1.23	7	207.01
25	1.54	8	236.58
30	1.85	9	266.16
35	2.16	10	295.73
40	2.46	11	325.30
45	2.77	12	354.88
50	3.08	13	384.45
55	3.39	14	414.02
60 (1 fl. dr.)	3.70	15	443.59
Fluid Drams		16 (1 pt.)	473.18
1	3.70	32 (1 qt.)	946.36
2	7.39	128 (1 gal.)	3785.43
3	11.09		
4	14.79		
5	18.48		
6	22.18		
7	25.88		
8 (1 fl. oz.)	29.57		

Weights/Measures

Metric—Avoirdupois Weight

Grams	Ounces
0.001 (1 mg.)	0.000035274
1	0.035274
1000 (kg.)	35.274 (2.2046 lb.)

Avoirdupois—Metric Weight

Ounces	Grams	
1/16	1.772	
1/8	3.544	
1/4	7.088	
1/2	14.175	
1	28.350	
2	56.699	
3	85.049	
4	113.398	
5	141.748	
6	170.097	
7	198.447	
8	226.796	
9	255.146	
10	283.495	
11	311.845	
12	340.194	
13	368.544	
14	396.893	
15	425.243	
16 (1 lb.)	453.59	
Pounds		
1 (16 oz.)	453.59	
2	907.18	
3	1360.78	(1.36 kg.)
4	1814.37	(1.81 kg.)
5	2267.96	(2.27 kg.)
6	2721.55	(2.72 kg.)
7	3175.15	(3.18 kg.)
8	3628.74	(3.63 kg.)
9	4082.33	(4.08 kg.)
10	4535.92	(4.54 kg.)

Apothecaries'—Metric and Metric—Apothecaries' Weight

Apothecaries'—Metric Weight		Metric—Apothecaries' Weight	
Grains	Grams	Milli-grams	Grains
1/150	0.0004	1	0.015432
1/120	0.0005	2	0.030864
1/100	0.0006	3	0.046296
1/80	0.0008	4	0.061728
1/64	0.001	5	0.077160
1/50	0.0013	6	0.092592
1/48	0.0014	7	0.108024
1/30	0.0022	8	0.123456
1/25	0.0026	9	0.138888
1/16	0.004	10	0.154320
1/12	0.005	15	0.231480
1/10	0.006	20	0.308640
1/9	0.007	25	0.385800
1/8	0.008	30	0.462960
1/7	0.009	35	0.540120
1/6	0.01	40	0.617280
1/5	0.013	45	0.694440
1/4	0.016	50	0.771600
1/3	0.02	100	1.543240
1/2	0.032		
1	0.065	**Grams**	
1 1/2	0.097 (0.1)	0.1	1.5432
2	0.125	0.2	3.0864
3	0.20	0.3	4.6296
4	0.25	0.4	6.1728
5	0.30	0.5	7.7160
6	0.40	0.6	9.2592
7	0.45	0.7	10.8024
8	0.50	0.8	12.3456
9	0.60	0.9	13.8888
10	0.65	1.0	15.4320

Continued

Apothecaries'—Metric and Metric—Apothecaries' Weight *(continued)*

Apothecaries'—Metric Weight		Metric—Apothecaries' Weight	
Grains	Grams	Milli-grams	Grains
15	1.00	1.5	23.1480
20 (1 ℈)	1.30	2.0	30.8640
30	2.00	2.5	38.5800
Scruples		3.0	46.2960
1	1.296 (1.3)	3.5	54.0120
2	2.592 (2.6)	4.0	61.728
3 (1 ʒ)	3.888 (3.9)	4.5	69.444
Drams		5.0	77.162
1	3.888	10.0	154.324
2	7.776		
3	11.664	**Equivalents**	
4	15.552	10	2.572 drams
5	19.440	15	3.858 drams
6	23.328	20	5.144 drams
7	27.216	25	6.430 drams
8 (1 ℥)	31.103	30	7.716 drams
Ounces		40	1.286 oz
1	31.103	45	1.447 oz
2	62.207	50	1.607 oz
3	93.310	100	3.215 oz
4	124.414	200	6.430 oz
5	155.517	300	9.644 oz
6	186.621	400	12.859 oz
7	217.724	500	1.34 lb
8	248.828	600	1.61 lb
9	279.931	700	1.88 lb
10	311.035	800	2.14 lb
11	342.138	900	2.41 lb
12 (1 lb)	373.242	1000	2.68 lb

From: Miller/Keane: Encyclopedia & Dictionary of Medicine, Nursing, & Allied Health (6th ed.). Philadelphia: WB Saunders, p.1797-1798. Reprinted with permission.

Table of Temperature Equivalents

Celsius (Centigrade) : Farenheit Scale

Celsius: Fahrenheit $°F = (°C × 9/5) + 32$				Fahrenheit: Celsius $°C = (°F — 32)× 5/9$			
°C	°F	°C	°F	°F	°C	°F	°C
−50	−58.0	49	120.2	−50	−46.7	99	37.2	157	69.4

Celsius: Fahrenheit — $°F = (°C × 9/5) + 32$				Fahrenheit: Celsius — $°C = (°F — 32) × 5/9$					
°C	°F	°C	°F	°F	°C	°F	°C	°F	°C
−50	−58.0	49	120.2	−50	−46.7	99	37.2	157	69.4
−40	−40.0	50	122.0	−40	−40.0	100	37.7	158	70.0
−35	−31.0	51	123.8	−35	−37.2	101	38.3	159	70.5
−30	−22.0	52	125.6	−30	−34.4	102	38.8	160	71.1
−25	−13.0	53	127.4	−25	−31.7	103	39.4	161	71.6
−20	−4.0	54	129.2	−20	−28.9	104	40.0	162	72.2
−15	+5.0	55	131.0	−15	−26.6	105	40.5	163	72.7
−10	14.0	56	132.8	−10	−23.3	106	41.1	164	73.3
−5	23.0	57	134.6	−5	−20.6	107	41.6	165	73.8
0	32.0	58	136.4	0	−17.7	108	42.2	166	74.4
+1	33.8	59	138.2	+1	−17.2	109	42.7	167	75.0
2	35.6	60	140.0	5	−15.0	110	43.3	168	75.5
3	37.4	61	141.8	10	−12.2	111	43.8	169	76.1
4	39.2	62	143.6	15	−9.4	112	44.4	170	76.6
5	41.0	63	145.4	20	−6.6	113	45.0	171	77.2
6	42.8	64	147.2	25	−3.8	114	45.5	172	77.7
7	44.6	65	149.0	30	−1.1	115	46.1	173	78.3
8	46.4	66	150.8	31	−0.5	116	46.6	174	78.8
9	48.2	67	152.6	32	0	117	47.2	175	79.4
10	50.0	68	154.4	33	+0.5	118	47.7	176	80.0
11	51.8	69	156.2	34	1.1	119	48.3	177	80.5
12	53.6	70	158.0	35	1.6	120	48.8	178	81.1
13	55.4	71	159.8	36	2.2	121	49.4	179	81.6
14	57.2	72	161.6	37	2.7	122	50.0	180	82.2
15	59.0	73	163.4	38	3.3	123	50.5	181	82.7
16	60.8	74	165.2	39	3.8	124	51.1	182	83.3
17	62.6	75	167.0	40	4.4	125	51.6	183	83.8
18	64.4	76	168.8	41	5.0	126	52.2	184	84.4
19	66.2	77	170.6	42	5.5	127	52.7	185	85.0
20	68.0	78	172.4	43	6.1	128	53.3	186	85.5
21	69.8	79	174.2	44	6.6	129	53.8	187	86.1
22	71.6	80	176.0	45	7.2	130	54.4	188	86.6
23	73.4	81	177.8	46	7.7	131	55.0	189	87.2
24	75.2	82	179.6	47	8.3	132	55.5	190	87.7
25	77.0	83	181.4	48	8.8	133	56.1	191	88.3
26	78.8	84	183.2	49	9.4	134	56.6	192	88.8
27	80.6	85	185.0	50	10.0	135	57.2	193	89.4
28	82.4	86	186.8	55	12.7	136	57.7	194	90.0
29	84.2	87	188.6	60	15.5	137	58.3	195	90.5
30	86.0	88	190.4	65	18.3	138	58.8	196	91.1
31	87.8	89	192.2	70	21.1	139	59.4	197	91.6
32	89.6	90	194.0	75	23.8	140	60.0	198	92.2
33	91.4	91	195.8	80	26.6	141	60.5	199	92.7
34	93.2	92	197.6	85	29.4	142	61.1	200	93.3
35	95.0	93	199.4	86	30.0	143	61.6	201	93.8
36	96.8	94	210.2	87	30.5	144	62.2	202	94.4
37	98.6	95	203.0	88	31.0	145	62.7	203	95.0
38	100.4	96	204.8	89	31.6	146	63.3	204	95.5
39	102.2	97	206.6	90	32.2	147	63.8	205	96.1
40	104.0	98	208.4	91	32.7	148	64.4	206	96.6
41	105.8	99	210.2	92	33.3	149	65.0	207	97.2
42	107.6	100	212.0	93	33.8	150	65.5	208	97.7
43	109.4	101	213.8	94	34.4	151	66.1	209	98.3
44	111.2	102	215.6	95	35.0	152	66.6	210	98.8
45	113.0	103	217.4	96	35.5	153	67.2	211	99.4
46	114.8	104	219.2	97	36.1	154	67.7	212	100.0
47	116.6	105	221.0	98	36.6	155	68.3	213	100.5
48	118.4	106	222.8	98.6	37.0	156	68.8	214	101.1

From: Miller/Keane: Encyclopedia & Dictionary of Medicine, Nursing, & Allied Health (6th ed.). Philadelphia: WB Saunders, p.1800. Reprinted with permission.

Measures of Mass

Avoirdupois Weight

Grains	Drams	Ounces	Pounds	Metric Equivalents, Grams
1	0.0366	0.0023	0.00014	0.0647989
27.34	1	0.0625	0.0039	1.772
437.5	16	1	0.0625	28.350
7000	256	16	1	453.5924277

Apothecaries Weight

Grains	Scruples ($\ni$)	Drams ($\mathfrak{Z}$)	Ounces ($\mathfrak{Z}$)	Pounds (lb)	Metric Equivalents, Grams
1	0.05	0.0167	0.0021	0.00017	0.0647989
20	1	0.333	0.042	0.0035	1.296
60	3	1	0.125	0.0104	3.888
480	24	8	1	0.0833	31.103
5760	288	96	12	1	373.24177

Troy Weight

Grains	Pennyweights	Ounces	Pounds	Metric Equivalents, Grams
1	0.042	0.002	0.00017	0.0647989
24	1	0.05	0.0042	1.555
480	20	1	0.083	31.103
5760	240	12	1	373.24177

Metric Weight

Micro-gram	Milli-gram	Centi-gram	Deci-gram	Gram	Deka-gram	Hecto-gram	Kilo-gram	Equivalents Avoir-dupois	Apothe-caries
1	–	–	–	–	–	–	–	0.000015 grains	
10^3	1	–	–	–	–	–	–	0.015432 grains	
10^4	10	1	–	–	–	–	–	0.154323 grains	
10^5	10^2	10	1	–	–	–	–	1.543235 grains	
10^6	10^3	10^2	10	1	–	–	–	15.432356 grains	
10^7	10^4	10^3	10^2	10	1	–	–	5.6438 dr	7.7162 scr
10^8	10^5	10^4	10^3	10^2	10	1	–	3.527 oz	3.215 oz
10^9	10^6	10^5	10^4	10^3	10^2	10	1	2.2046 lb	2.6792 lb
10^{12}	10^9	10^8	10^7	10^6	10^5	10^4	10^3	2204.6223 lb	2679.2285 lb

From: Miller/Keane: Encyclopedia & Dictionary of Medicine, Nursing, & Allied Health (6th ed.). Philadelphia: WB Saunders, p.1795. Reprinted with permission.

Measures of Capacity

Apothecaries (Wine) Measure

Minims	Fluid Drams	Fluid Ounces	Gills	Pints	Quarts	Gallons	Cubic Inches	Milliliters	Cubic Centimeters
1	0.0166	0.002	0.0005	0.00013	—	—	0.00376	0.06161	0.06161
60	1	0.125	0.0312	0.0078	0.0039	—	0.22558	3.6967	3.6967
480	8	1	0.25	0.0625	0.0312	0.0078	1.80468	29.5737	29.5737
1920	32	4	1	0.25	0.125	0.0312	7.21875	118.2948	118.2948
7680	128	16	4	1	0.5	0.125	28.875	473.179	473.179
15360	256	32	8	2	1	0.25	57.75	946.358	946.358
61440	1024	128	32	8	4	1	231	3785.434	3785.434

From: Miller/Keane: Encyclopedia & Dictionary of Medicine, Nursing, & Allied Health (6th ed.). Philadelphia: WB Saunders, p.1795. Reprinted with permission.

Weights/Measures

Measures of Capacity

Metric Measure

Microliter	Milliliter	Centiliter	Deciliter	Liter	Dekaliter	Hectoliter	Kiloliter	Myrialiter	Equivalents (Apothecaries' Fluid)	
1	—	—	—	—	—	—	—	—	0.01623108	minim
10^3	1	—	—	—	—	—	—	—	16.23	minims
10^4	10	1	—	—	—	—	—	—	2.7	fluid drams
10^5	10^2	10	1	—	—	—	—	—	3.38	fluid ounces
10^6	10^3	10^2	10	1	—	—	—	—	2.11	pints
10^7	10^4	10^3	10^2	10	1	—	—	—	2.64	gallons
10^8	10^5	10^4	10^3	10^2	10	1	—	—	26.418	gallons
10^9	10^6	10^5	10^4	10^3	10^2	10	1	—	264.18	gallons
10^{10}	10^7	10^6	10^5	10^4	10^3	10^2	10	1	2641.8	gallons

1 liter = 2.113363738 pints (Apothecaries').

From: Miller/Keane: Encyclopedia & Dictionary of Medicine, Nursing, & Allied Health (6th ed.). Philadelphia: WB Saunders, p.1796. Reprinted with permission.

Weights/Measures

Measures of Length

Metric Measure

Micro-meter	Milli-meter	Centi-meter	Deci-meter	Meter	Deka-meter	Hecto-meter	Kilo-meter	Myria-meter	Mega-meter	Equivalents
1	0.001	10^{-4}	–	–	–	–	–	–	–	0.000039 inch
10^3	1	10^{-1}	–	–	–	–	–	–	–	0.03937 inch
10^4	10	1	–	–	–	–	–	–	–	0.3937 inch
10^5	10^2	10	1	–	–	–	–	–	–	3.937 inches
10^6	10^3	10^2	10	1	–	–	–	–	–	39.37 inches
10^7	10^4	10^3	10^2	10	1	–	–	–	–	10.9361 yards
10^8	10^5	10^4	10^3	10^2	10	1	–	–	–	109.3612 yards
10^9	10^6	10^5	10^4	10^3	10^2	10	1	–	–	1093.6121 yards
10^{10}	10^7	10^6	10^5	10^4	10^3	10^2	10	1	–	6.2137 miles
10^{12}	10^9	10^8	10^7	10^6	10^5	10^4	10^3	10^2	1	621.37 miles

From: Miller/Keane: Encyclopedia & Dictionary of Medicine, Nursing, & Allied Health (6th ed.). Philadelphia: WB Saunders, p.1796. Reprinted with permission.

Weights/Measures

How the Metric System Works

Type of Measurement	Units of Measurement	How it Compares With the US System
Length or Distance	*meter* (m) = basic unit	A little more than 1 yard (1 yard = 36 inches and 1 meter = 39.37 inches)
	millimeter (mm) = 0.001 meter	About the size of the width of a pinhead. There are just over 25 millimeters in 1 inch.
	centimeter (cm) = 0.01 meter	About 2/5 (or 0.4) of an inch, the width of a child's little finger. There are about 2 1/2 centimeters in an inch.
	decimeter (dm) = 0.1 meter	About 4 inches
	dekameter (dam) = 10 meters	A little more than 10 yards
	hectometer (hm) = 100 meters	A little more than 100 yards
	kilometer (km) = 1000 meters	About 3/5 (or 0.62) of a mile
Liquids or Volume	*liter* (L) = basic unit	Approximately 1 quart (2 liters is now a popular-sized soft drink bottle; that's about 1/2 gallon because there are 4 quarts in a gallon)
	*milliliter** (mL) = 0.001 liter	*Very* small drop (commonly used in medicine)
	centiliter (cL) = 0.01 liter	About 2 teaspoons
	deciliter (dL) = 0.1 liter	Between 1/3 and 1/2 cup
	dekaliter (daL) = 10 liters	About 10 quarts or 2 1/2 gallons
	hectoliter (hL) = 100 liters	About 25 gallons
	kiloliter (kL) = 1000 liters	About 250 gallons

Continued

How the Metric System Works *(continued)*

Type of Measurement	Units of Measurement	How it Compares With the US System
Weight or Mass of Solids	*gram* (Gm, g) = basic unit	Approximately 1/28 of an ounce. About the weight of a paperclip.
	microgram (mcg) = 0.000001 gram	An incredibly small amount (1 millionth of 1/400 of a pound!) Don't be fooled, however. This can be a significant amount in health care. The body depends on very small quantities of certain substances to function properly. It can also be harmed by minute amounts of the wrong substances.
	milligram (mg) = 0.001 gram	Also very small amounts, although they are many times heavier than a microgram.
	centigram (cg) = 0.01 gram	
	decigram (dg) = 0.1 gram	
	dekagram (dag) = 10 grams	5/14 of an ounce
	hectogram (hg) = 100 grams	About 3 1/2 ounces
	kilogram (kg) = 1000 grams	2.2 pounds

Continued

Weights/Measures

How the Metric System Works *(continued)*

Weights/Measures

Type of Measurement	Units of Measurement	How it Compares With the US System
Temperature	Celsius (commonly called centigrade) 0° C = freezing point of water 100° C = boiling point of water	Fahrenheit is the system commonly used in the United States. In this system, 32° F is freezing and 95° F is a sunny day at the beach.
	Celsius thermometers are marked in one-tenth intervals.	1° C = 1.8 times 1° F
	Water freezes: 0° C	32° F
	Normal body temperature: 37° C	98.6° F
	Water boils: 100° C	212° F
	Sterilization occurs: 121° C	250° F
	To convert between the 2 systems:	
	Fahrenheit to Celsius: 1. Subtract 32 from the F temperature 2. Multiply by 5/9	98.6° F 98.6 − 32 = 66.6 5/9 × 66.6 = 5/9 × 66.6/1.0 = 37
	Celsius to Fahrenheit: 1. Multiply the C temperature by 9/5 2. Add 32	37 × 9/5 = 37/1 × 9/5 = 333/5 = 66.6 66.6 + 32 = 98.6

*A milliliter is the same amount as a cubic centimeter (cc). This is important to know in health care because these terms are sometimes used interchangeably.

From: Haroun, L. (2000). Career Development for Health Professionals Phila.: W B Saunders, p. 146-147, Table 6-3. Reprinted with permission.

PROGRAM OVERVIEW

Program Name: _____
Credits/Units/Hours Needed: _____ Estimated Graduation: _____
Guidance Counselor: _____ Phone: _____

Course	Completed	Instructor	Credits/ Units/ Hours	Date/Time of Course Other Notes

Planner—Overview

TERM/SEMESTER OVERVIEW

Term/Semester: _____

Credits/Units/Hours Total: _____ Estimated Graduation: _____

Guidance Counselor: _____ Phone: _____

Course	Credits/ Units/ Hours	Instructor	Phone	Course Date/ Time	Notes

TERM / SEMESTER OVERVIEW

Term/Semester: _____

Credits/Units/Hours Total: _____ Estimated Graduation: _____

Guidance Counselor: _____ Phone: _____

Course	Credits/ Units/ Hours	Instructor	Phone	Course Date/ Time	Notes

Planner—Overview

TERM/SEMESTER OVERVIEW

Term/Semester: _____
Credits/Units/Hours Total: _____ Estimated Graduation: _____
Guidance Counselor: _____ Phone: _____

Course	Credits/ Units/ Hours	Instructor	Phone	Course Date/ Time	Notes

COURSE OVERVIEW

Course Name: _____ Course #: _____
Credits/Units/Hours: _____ Location: _____
Instructor: _____ Phone: _____
Lab: Y N Lab Location: _____ Lab Days/Times: _____
Study Partner(s): _____
_____
Texts/Materials: _____
Test Dates: _____

Assignment	Due Date	Completed	Notes

Planner—Overview

COURSE OVERVIEW

Course Name: _____ Course #: _____
Credits/Units/Hours: _____ Location: _____
Instructor: _____ Phone: _____
Lab: Y N Lab Location: _____ Lab Days/Times: _____
Study Partner(s): _____
_____
Texts/Materials: _____
Test Dates: _____

Planner—Overview

Assignment	Due Date	Completed	Notes

COURSE OVERVIEW

Course Name: _____ Course #: _____
Credits/Units/Hours: _____ Location: _____
Instructor: _____ Phone: _____
Lab: Y   N   Lab Location: _____ Lab Days/Times: _____
Study Partner(s): _____
_____

Texts/Materials: _____
Test Dates: _____

Assignment	Due Date	Completed	Notes

COURSE OVERVIEW

Course Name: _____ Course #: _____
Credits/Units/Hours: _____ Location: _____
Instructor: _____ Phone: _____
Lab: Y N Lab Location: _____ Lab Days/Times: _____
Study Partner(s): _____
_____

Texts/Materials: _____
Test Dates: _____

Assignment	Due Date	Completed	Notes

COURSE OVERVIEW

Course Name: _____ Course #: _____
Credits/Units/Hours: _____ Location: _____
Instructor: _____ Phone: _____
Lab: Y N Lab Location: _____ Lab Days/Times: _____
Study Partner(s): _____
_____
Texts/Materials: _____
Test Dates: _____

Assignment	Due Date	Completed	Notes

Planner—Overview

COURSE OVERVIEW

Course Name: _____   Course #: _____
Credits/Units/Hours: _____   Location: _____
Instructor: _____   Phone: _____
Lab: Y N Lab Location: _____   Lab Days/Times: _____
Study Partner(s): _____
_____

Texts/Materials: _____
Test Dates: _____

Assignment	Due Date	Completed	Notes

COURSE OVERVIEW

Course Name: _____ Course #: _____
Credits/Units/Hours: _____ Location: _____
Instructor: _____ Phone: _____
Lab: Y N Lab Location: _____ Lab Days/Times: _____
Study Partner(s): _____
_____
Texts/Materials: _____
Test Dates: _____

Assignment	Due Date	Completed	Notes

COURSE OVERVIEW

Course Name: _____ Course #: _____

Credits/Units/Hours: _____ Location: _____

Instructor: _____ Phone: _____

Lab: Y N Lab Location: _____ Lab Days/Times: _____

Study Partner(s): _____

_____

Texts/Materials: _____

Test Dates: _____

Assignment	Due Date	Completed	Notes

COURSE ASSIGNMENTS

Term or Semester: _____

Date of Assignment Due or Test	Assignment or Test	C O M P L E T E D	Course	Description	Importance (% of grade)	Notes
	A T					
	A T					
	A T					
	A T					
	A T					
	A T					
	A T					
	A T					

COURSE ASSIGNMENTS

Term or Semester: _____

Date of Assignment Due or Test	Assignment or Test	C O M P L E T E D	Course	Description	Importance (% of grade)	Notes
	A T					
	A T					
	A T					
	A T					
	A T					
	A T					
	A T					
	A T					

COURSE ASSIGNMENTS

Term or Semester: _____

Date of Assignment Due or Test	Assignment or Test	C O M P L E T E D	Course	Description	Importance (% of grade)	Notes
	A T					
	A T					
	A T					
	A T					
	A T					
	A T					
	A T					
	A T					

COURSE ASSIGNMENTS

Term or Semester: _____

Date of Assignment Due or Test	Assignment or Test	C O M P L E T E D	Course	Description	Importance (% of grade)	Notes
	A T					
	A T					
	A T					
	A T					
	A T					
	A T					
	A T					
	A T					

COURSE ASSIGNMENTS

Term or Semester: _____

Date of Assignment Due or Test	Assignment or Test	C O M P L E T E D	Course	Description	Importance (% of grade)	Notes
	A T					
	A T					
	A T					
	A T					
	A T					
	A T					
	A T					
	A T					

COURSE ASSIGNMENTS

Term or Semester: _____

Date of Assignment Due or Test	Assignment or Test	COMPLETED	Course	Description	Importance (% of grade)	Notes
	A T					
	A T					
	A T					
	A T					
	A T					
	A T					
	A T					
	A T					

BIG GOAL FORM

Completion Date
Exact or Approximate

Goal:

WHY this goal is worth the time & effort:

WHAT it will take (Action Steps):	*DEADLINE* for each
1.	
2.	
3.	
4.	
Other:	

RESOURCES I need:	*Check* when secured

VISUALIZATION/AFFIRMATION statement of goal:

Commitment Statement and Signature:
I accept this goal and agree to the action steps necessary to reach this
goal by _____ (date).

_____
Signature

Clip when complete
See other side for Notes ➡

BIG GOAL NOTES:

Planner—Overview

_____
_____
_____
_____
_____
_____
_____
_____
_____
_____
_____
_____
_____
_____
_____
_____
_____
_____
_____
_____
_____
_____
_____
_____
_____
_____
_____
_____
_____

BIG GOAL FORM

Completion Date
Exact or Approximate

Goal:

WHY this goal is worth the time & effort:

WHAT it will take (Action Steps):	DEADLINE for each
1.	
2.	
3.	
4.	
Other:	

RESOURCES I need:	Check when secured

VISUALIZATION/AFFIRMATION statement of goal:

Commitment Statement and Signature:
I accept this goal and agree to the action steps necessary to reach this goal by _____ (date).

_____
Signature

Clip when complete
See other side for Notes ➡

BIG GOAL NOTES:

BIG GOAL FORM

Completion Date
Exact or Approximate

Goal:

WHY this goal is worth the time & effort:

WHAT it will take (Action Steps):	**DEADLINE** for each
1.	
2.	
3.	
4.	
Other:	

RESOURCES I need:	**Check** when secured

VISUALIZATION/AFFIRMATION statement of goal:

Commitment Statement and Signature:
I accept this goal and agree to the action steps necessary to reach this
goal by _____ (date).

_____
Signature

Clip when complete
See other side for Notes ➡

BIG GOAL NOTES:

Planner—Overview

BIG GOAL FORM

Completion Date
Exact or Approximate

Goal:

WHY this goal is worth the time & effort:

WHAT it will take (Action Steps):	**DEADLINE** *for each*
1.	
2.	
3.	
4.	
Other:	

RESOURCES I need:	**Check** *when secured*

VISUALIZATION/AFFIRMATION statement of goal:

Commitment Statement and Signature:
I accept this goal and agree to the action steps necessary to reach this
goal by _____ (date).

_____
Signature

Clip when complete
See other side for Notes ➡

BIG GOAL NOTES:

BIG GOAL FORM

Completion Date
Exact or Approximate

Goal:

WHY this goal is worth the time & effort:

WHAT it will take (Action Steps):	**DEADLINE** for each
1.	
2.	
3.	
4.	
Other:	

RESOURCES I need:	**Check** when secured

VISUALIZATION/AFFIRMATION statement of goal:

Commitment Statement and Signature:
I accept this goal and agree to the action steps necessary to reach this
goal by _____ (date).

_____
Signature

Clip when complete
See other side for Notes ➡

BIG GOAL NOTES:

Monthly Planning Section

Date Calendar for 2005—2008 and 12 Monthly Planning Forms

Clip off the corners of the Monthly Planning Forms after the month is over. Your calendar will open easily to the current month.

2005

January

S	M	T	W	T	F	S
						1
2	3	4	5	6	7	8
9	10	11	12	13	14	15
16	17	18	19	20	21	22
23	24	25	26	27	28	29
30	31					

February

S	M	T	W	T	F	S
		1	2	3	4	5
6	7	8	9	10	11	12
13	14	15	16	17	18	19
20	21	22	23	24	25	26
27	28					

March

S	M	T	W	T	F	S
		1	2	3	4	5
6	7	8	9	10	11	12
13	14	15	16	17	18	19
20	21	22	23	24	25	26
27	28	29	30	31		

April

S	M	T	W	T	F	S
					1	2
3	4	5	6	7	8	9
10	11	12	13	14	15	16
17	18	19	20	21	22	23
24	25	26	27	28	29	30

May

S	M	T	W	T	F	S
1	2	3	4	5	6	7
8	9	10	11	12	13	14
15	16	17	18	19	20	21
22	23	24	25	26	27	28
29	30	31				

June

S	M	T	W	T	F	S
			1	2	3	4
5	6	7	8	9	10	11
12	13	14	15	16	17	18
19	20	21	22	23	24	25
26	27	28	29	30		

July

S	M	T	W	T	F	S
					1	2
3	4	5	6	7	8	9
10	11	12	13	14	15	16
17	18	19	20	21	22	23
24	25	26	27	28	29	30
31						

August

S	M	T	W	T	F	S
	1	2	3	4	5	6
7	8	9	10	11	12	13
14	15	16	17	18	19	20
21	22	23	24	25	26	27
28	29	30	31			

September

S	M	T	W	T	F	S
				1	2	3
4	5	6	7	8	9	10
11	12	13	14	15	16	17
18	19	20	21	22	23	24
25	26	27	28	29	30	

October

S	M	T	W	T	F	S
						1
2	3	4	5	6	7	8
9	10	11	12	13	14	15
16	17	18	19	20	21	22
23	24	25	26	27	28	29
30	31					

November

S	M	T	W	T	F	S
		1	2	3	4	5
6	7	8	9	10	11	12
13	14	15	16	17	18	19
20	21	22	23	24	25	26
27	28	29	30			

December

S	M	T	W	T	F	S
				1	2	3
4	5	6	7	8	9	10
11	12	13	14	15	16	17
18	19	20	21	22	23	24
25	26	27	28	29	30	31

2006

January

S	M	T	W	T	F	S
1	2	3	4	5	6	7
8	9	10	11	12	13	14
15	16	17	18	19	20	21
22	23	24	25	26	27	28
29	30	31				

February

S	M	T	W	T	F	S
			1	2	3	4
5	6	7	8	9	10	11
12	13	14	15	16	17	18
19	20	21	22	23	24	25
26	27	28				

March

S	M	T	W	T	F	S
			1	2	3	4
5	6	7	8	9	10	11
12	13	14	15	16	17	18
19	20	21	22	23	24	25
26	27	28	29	30	31	

April

S	M	T	W	T	F	S
						1
2	3	4	5	6	7	8
9	10	11	12	13	14	15
16	17	18	19	20	21	22
23	24	25	26	27	28	29
30						

May

S	M	T	W	T	F	S
	1	2	3	4	5	6
7	8	9	10	11	12	13
14	15	16	17	18	19	20
21	22	23	24	25	26	27
28	29	30	31			

June

S	M	T	W	T	F	S
				1	2	3
4	5	6	7	8	9	10
11	12	13	14	15	16	17
18	19	20	21	22	23	24
25	26	27	28	29	30	

July

S	M	T	W	T	F	S
						1
2	3	4	5	6	7	8
9	10	11	12	13	14	15
16	17	18	19	20	21	22
23	24	25	26	27	28	29
30	31					

August

S	M	T	W	T	F	S
		1	2	3	4	5
6	7	8	9	10	11	12
13	14	15	16	17	18	19
20	21	22	23	24	25	26
27	28	29	30	31		

September

S	M	T	W	T	F	S
					1	2
3	4	5	6	7	8	9
10	11	12	13	14	15	16
17	18	19	20	21	22	23
24	25	26	27	28	29	30

October

S	M	T	W	T	F	S
1	2	3	4	5	6	7
8	9	10	11	12	13	14
15	16	17	18	19	20	21
22	23	24	25	26	27	28
29	30	31				

November

S	M	T	W	T	F	S
			1	2	3	4
5	6	7	8	9	10	11
12	13	14	15	16	17	18
19	20	21	22	23	24	25
26	27	28	29	30		

December

S	M	T	W	T	F	S
					1	2
3	4	5	6	7	8	9
10	11	12	13	14	15	16
17	18	19	20	21	22	23
24	25	26	27	28	29	30
31						

2007

January
S	M	T	W	T	F	S
	1	2	3	4	5	6
7	8	9	10	11	12	13
14	15	16	17	18	19	20
21	22	23	24	25	26	27
28	29	30	31			

February
S	M	T	W	T	F	S
				1	2	3
4	5	6	7	8	9	10
11	12	13	14	15	16	17
18	19	20	21	22	23	24
25	26	27	28			

March
S	M	T	W	T	F	S
				1	2	3
4	5	6	7	8	9	10
11	12	13	14	15	16	17
18	19	20	21	22	23	24
25	26	27	28	29	30	31

April
S	M	T	W	T	F	S
1	2	3	4	5	6	7
8	9	10	11	12	13	14
15	16	17	18	19	20	21
22	23	24	25	26	27	28
29	30					

May
S	M	T	W	T	F	S
		1	2	3	4	5
6	7	8	9	10	11	12
13	14	15	16	17	18	19
20	21	22	23	24	25	26
27	28	29	30	31		

June
S	M	T	W	T	F	S
					1	2
3	4	5	6	7	8	9
10	11	12	13	14	15	16
17	18	19	20	21	22	23
24	25	26	27	28	29	30

July
S	M	T	W	T	F	S
1	2	3	4	5	6	7
8	9	10	11	12	13	14
15	16	17	18	19	20	21
22	23	24	25	26	27	28
29	30	31				

August
S	M	T	W	T	F	S
			1	2	3	4
5	6	7	8	9	10	11
12	13	14	15	16	17	18
19	20	21	22	23	24	25
26	27	28	29	30	31	

September
S	M	T	W	T	F	S
						1
2	3	4	5	6	7	8
9	10	11	12	13	14	15
16	17	18	19	20	21	22
23	24	25	26	27	28	29
30						

October
S	M	T	W	T	F	S
	1	2	3	4	5	6
7	8	9	10	11	12	13
14	15	16	17	18	19	20
21	22	23	24	25	26	27
28	29	30	31			

November
S	M	T	W	T	F	S
				1	2	3
4	5	6	7	8	9	10
11	12	13	14	15	16	17
18	19	20	21	22	23	24
25	26	27	28	29	30	

December
S	M	T	W	T	F	S
						1
2	3	4	5	6	7	8
9	10	11	12	13	14	15
16	17	18	19	20	21	22
23	24	25	26	27	28	29
30	31					

2008

January
S	M	T	W	T	F	S
		1	2	3	4	5
6	7	8	9	10	11	12
13	14	15	16	17	18	19
20	21	22	23	24	25	26
27	28	29	30	31		

February
S	M	T	W	T	F	S
					1	2
3	4	5	6	7	8	9
10	11	12	13	14	15	16
17	18	19	20	21	22	23
24	25	26	27	28	29	

March
S	M	T	W	T	F	S
						1
2	3	4	5	6	7	8
9	10	11	12	13	14	15
16	17	18	19	20	21	22
23	24	25	26	27	28	29
30	31					

April
S	M	T	W	T	F	S
		1	2	3	4	5
6	7	8	9	10	11	12
13	14	15	16	17	18	19
20	21	22	23	24	25	26
27	28	29	30			

May
S	M	T	W	T	F	S
				1	2	3
4	5	6	7	8	9	10
11	12	13	14	15	16	17
18	19	20	21	22	23	24
25	26	27	28	29	30	31

June
S	M	T	W	T	F	S
1	2	3	4	5	6	7
8	9	10	11	12	13	14
15	16	17	18	19	20	21
22	23	24	25	26	27	28
29	30					

July
S	M	T	W	T	F	S
		1	2	3	4	5
6	7	8	9	10	11	12
13	14	15	16	17	18	19
20	21	22	23	24	25	26
27	28	29	30	31		

August
S	M	T	W	T	F	S
					1	2
3	4	5	6	7	8	9
10	11	12	13	14	15	16
17	18	19	20	21	22	23
24	25	26	27	28	29	30
31						

September
S	M	T	W	T	F	S
	1	2	3	4	5	6
7	8	9	10	11	12	13
14	15	16	17	18	19	20
21	22	23	24	25	26	27
28	29	30				

October
S	M	T	W	T	F	S
			1	2	3	4
5	6	7	8	9	10	11
12	13	14	15	16	17	18
19	20	21	22	23	24	25
26	27	28	29	30	31	

November
S	M	T	W	T	F	S
						1
2	3	4	5	6	7	8
9	10	11	12	13	14	15
16	17	18	19	20	21	22
23	24	25	26	27	28	29
30						

December
S	M	T	W	T	F	S
	1	2	3	4	5	6
7	8	9	10	11	12	13
14	15	16	17	18	19	20
21	22	23	24	25	26	27
28	29	30	31			

Month:

Goals for the Month:

Monday	Tuesday	Wednesday

Notes:

Thursday	Friday	Saturday/Sunday

Clip for current month ➡

Planner—Monthly

Month:

Goals for the Month:

Monday	Tuesday	Wednesday

← Clip for current month

Notes:

Thursday	Friday	Saturday/Sunday

Clip for current month ➡

Month:

Goals for the Month:

Monday	Tuesday	Wednesday

← Clip for current month

Notes:

Thursday	Friday	Saturday/Sunday

Clip for current month ➡

Month:

Goals for the Month:

Monday	Tuesday	Wednesday

← Clip for current month

Notes:

Thursday	Friday	Saturday/Sunday

Month:

Goals for the Month:

Monday	Tuesday	Wednesday

Planner—Monthly

← Clip for current month

Notes:

Thursday	Friday	Saturday/Sunday

Month:

Goals for the Month:

Monday	Tuesday	Wednesday

← Clip for current month

Notes:

Thursday	Friday	Saturday/Sunday

Clip for current month ➡

Month:

Goals for the Month:

Monday	Tuesday	Wednesday

Planner—Monthly

← Clip for current month

Notes:

Thursday	Friday	Saturday/Sunday

Clip for current month ➡

Month:

Goals for the Month:

Monday	Tuesday	Wednesday

Planner—Monthly

← Clip for current month

Notes:

Thursday	Friday	Saturday/Sunday

Clip for current month →

Month:

Goals for the Month:

Monday	Tuesday	Wednesday

← Clip for current month

Notes:

Thursday	Friday	Saturday/Sunday

Clip for current month ➡

Planner—Monthly

Month:

Goals for the Month:

Monday	Tuesday	Wednesday

← Clip for current month

Notes:

Thursday	Friday	Saturday/Sunday

Clip for current month ➡

Month:

Goals for the Month:

Monday	Tuesday	Wednesday

← Clip for current month

Notes:

Thursday	Friday	Saturday/Sunday

Clip for current month ➡

Month:

Goals for the Month:

Planner—Monthly

Monday	Tuesday	Wednesday

← Clip for current month

Notes:

Thursday	Friday	Saturday/Sunday

Clip for current month ➜

52 Weekly Plan Forms

Clip off the corners of the Weekly Plan Forms after the week is over. Your calendar will open easily to the current week.

Planner—Weekly

Clip for current week ➔

Week of: _____

Goals for the Week: *Study all 4 Lectures of Transitions, Try to exercise*

Monday

Tuesday

Wednesday

Notes:

Thursday
① finish chap 1A Fundementals 5
② Get House organized
③ Stretch hip exercise
④ Review chap 4 friends notes ✓
   Check Guidelines on 4 From Excelsior ✓
⑤ Ck account For Bal Money
⑥ send fax to State Farm
⑦ Remind Connor To call State Farm ✓

Friday

Saturday/Sunday

Week of: _____

Goals for the Week:

Monday

Tuesday

Wednesday

← Clip for current week

Notes:

Thursday

Friday

Saturday/Sunday

Clip for current week ➡

Week of: _____

Goals for the Week:

Monday

Tuesday

Wednesday

← Clip for current week

Notes:

Thursday

Friday

Saturday/Sunday

Planner—Weekly

Clip for current week ➡

Week of: _____

Goals for the Week:

Monday

Tuesday

Wednesday

← Clip for current week

Notes:

Thursday

Friday

Saturday/Sunday

Planner—Weekly

Clip for current week ➡

Week of: _____

Goals for the Week:

Monday

Tuesday

Wednesday

← Clip for current week

Notes:

Thursday

Friday

Saturday/Sunday

Clip for current week ➡

Week of: _____

Goals for the Week:

Monday

Tuesday

Wednesday

Notes:

Thursday

Friday

Saturday/Sunday

Clip for current week ➜

Week of: _____

Goals for the Week:

Monday

Tuesday

Wednesday

← Clip for current week

Notes:

Thursday

Friday

Saturday/Sunday

Clip for current week ➡

Week of: _____

Goals for the Week:

Monday

Tuesday

Wednesday

← Clip for current week

Notes:

Thursday

Friday

Saturday/Sunday

Clip for current week ➡

Week of: _____

Goals for the Week:

Monday

Tuesday

Wednesday

← Clip for current week

Notes:

Thursday

Friday

Saturday/Sunday

Clip for current week ➡

Week of: _____

Goals for the Week:

Monday

Tuesday

Wednesday

← Clip for current week

Notes:

Thursday

Friday

Saturday/Sunday

Clip for current week ➡

Week of: _____

Goals for the Week:

Monday

Tuesday

Wednesday

← Clip for current week

Notes:

Thursday

Friday

Saturday/Sunday

Clip for current week ➡

Week of: _____

Goals for the Week:

Monday

Tuesday

Wednesday

← Clip for current week

Notes:

Thursday

Friday

Saturday/Sunday

Clip for current week ➜

Week of: _____

Goals for the Week:

Monday

Tuesday

Wednesday

← Clip for current week

Notes:

Thursday

Friday

Saturday/Sunday

Clip for current week ➡

Week of: _____

Goals for the Week:

Monday

Tuesday

Wednesday

← Clip for current week

Notes:

Thursday

Friday

Saturday/Sunday

Clip for current week ➡

Week of: _____

Goals for the Week:

Monday

Tuesday

Wednesday

← Clip for current week

Notes:

Thursday

Friday

Saturday/Sunday

Clip for current week →

Week of: _____

Goals for the Week:

Monday

Tuesday

Wednesday

← Clip for current week

Notes:

Thursday

Friday

Saturday/Sunday

Clip for current week ➡

Week of: _____

Goals for the Week:

Monday

Tuesday

Wednesday

← Clip for current week

Notes:

Thursday

Friday

Saturday/Sunday

Clip for current week ➜

Week of: _____

Goals for the Week:

Monday

Tuesday

Wednesday

← Clip for current week

Planner—Weekly

Notes:

Thursday

Friday

Saturday/Sunday

Clip for current week ➡

Week of: _____

Goals for the Week:

Monday

Tuesday

Wednesday

← Clip for current week

Notes:

Thursday

Friday

Saturday/Sunday

Clip for current week ➡

Week of: _____

Goals for the Week:

Monday

Tuesday

Wednesday

← Clip for current week

Notes:

Thursday

Friday

Saturday/Sunday

Clip for current week ➡

Week of: _____

Goals for the Week:

Monday

Tuesday

Wednesday

← Clip for current week

Notes:

Thursday

Friday

Saturday/Sunday

Clip for current week ➡

Week of: _____

Goals for the Week:

Monday

Tuesday

Wednesday

← Clip for current week

Notes:

Thursday

Friday

Saturday/Sunday

Clip for current week ➡

Week of: _____

Planner—Weekly

Goals for the Week:

Monday

Tuesday

Wednesday

← Clip for current week

Notes:

Thursday

Friday

Saturday/Sunday

Clip for current week ➤

Week of: _____

Goals for the Week:

Monday

Tuesday

Wednesday

← Clip for current week

Notes:

Thursday

Friday

Saturday/Sunday

Clip for current week ➡

Week of: _____

Goals for the Week:

Monday

Tuesday

Wednesday

← Clip for current week

Notes:

Thursday

Friday

Saturday/Sunday

Clip for current week ➡

Week of: _____

Goals for the Week:

Monday

Tuesday

Wednesday

← Clip for current week

Notes:

Thursday

Friday

Saturday/Sunday

Clip for current week ➡

Week of: _____

Goals for the Week:

Monday

Tuesday

Wednesday

← Clip for current week

Notes:

Thursday

Friday

Saturday/Sunday

Clip for current week ➡

Week of: _____

Goals for the Week:

Monday

Tuesday

Wednesday

← Clip for current week

Notes:

Thursday

Friday

Saturday/Sunday

Clip for current week ➡

Week of: _____

Goals for the Week:

Monday

Tuesday

Wednesday

← Clip for current week

Notes:

Thursday

Friday

Saturday/Sunday

Clip for current week ➜

Week of: _____

Goals for the Week:

Monday

Tuesday

Wednesday

← Clip for current week

Notes:

Thursday

Friday

Saturday/Sunday

Clip for current week ➡

Week of: _____

Goals for the Week:

Monday

Tuesday

Wednesday

← Clip for current week

Notes:

Thursday

Friday

Saturday/Sunday

Clip for current week ➜

Week of: _____

Goals for the Week:

Monday ☐

Tuesday ☐

Wednesday ☐

Planner—Weekly

← Clip for current week

Notes:

Thursday

Friday

Saturday/Sunday

Clip for current week ➡

Week of: _____

Goals for the Week:

Monday

Tuesday

Wednesday

← Clip for current week

Notes:

Thursday

Friday

Saturday/Sunday

Clip for current week ➡

Week of: _____

Goals for the Week:

Monday

Tuesday

Wednesday

← Clip for current week

Notes:

Thursday

Friday

Saturday/Sunday

Clip for current week ➡

Week of: _____

Goals for the Week:

Monday

Tuesday

Wednesday

← Clip for current week

1126

Notes:

365

Thursday

$\frac{2}{3}$ ($\frac{4}{6}$

$\div \frac{2}{2}$ $\frac{6}{6}$ 1

Friday

600.00 ALL WTL

= 1200

POD 2 Rooms

Saturday/Sunday

1485
850

635.00

Week of: _____

Goals for the Week:

Monday ☐

Tuesday ☐

Wednesday ☐

Planner—Weekly

← Clip for current week

Notes:

Thursday

Friday

Saturday/Sunday

Clip for current week ➡

Week of: _____

Goals for the Week:

Monday

Tuesday

Wednesday

← Clip for current week

Notes:

Thursday

Friday

Saturday/Sunday

Clip for current week ➡

Week of: _____

Goals for the Week:

Monday

Tuesday

Wednesday

← Clip for current week

Notes:

Thursday

Friday

Saturday/Sunday

Clip for current week ➡

Week of: _____

Goals for the Week:

Monday ☐

Tuesday ☐

Wednesday ☐

Planner—Weekly

← Clip for current week

Notes:

Thursday

Friday

Saturday/Sunday

Clip for current week ➡

Week of: _____

Goals for the Week:

Monday

Tuesday

Wednesday

← Clip for current week

Notes:

Thursday

Friday

Saturday/Sunday

Clip for current week ➡

Week of: _____

Goals for the Week:

Monday	

Tuesday	

Wednesday	

← Clip for current week

Notes:

Thursday

Friday

Saturday/Sunday

Clip for current week ➡

Week of: _____

Goals for the Week:

Monday

Tuesday

Wednesday

Notes:

Thursday

Friday

Saturday/Sunday

Planner—Weekly

Clip for current week ➡

Week of: _____

Goals for the Week:

Monday

Tuesday

Wednesday

← Clip for current week

Notes:

Thursday

Friday

Saturday/Sunday

Clip for current week ➡

Week of: _____

Goals for the Week:

Monday

Tuesday

Wednesday

← Clip for current week

Notes:

Thursday

Friday

Saturday/Sunday

Clip for current week ➡

Week of: _____

Goals for the Week:

Monday

Tuesday

Wednesday

← Clip for current week

Notes:

Thursday

Friday

Saturday/Sunday

Clip for current week ➡

Week of: _____

Goals for the Week:

Monday

Tuesday

Wednesday

← Clip for current week

Notes:

Thursday

Friday

Saturday/Sunday

Clip for current week ➜

Week of: _____

Goals for the Week:

Monday

Tuesday

Wednesday

← Clip for current week

Notes:

Thursday

Friday

Saturday/Sunday

Clip for current week ➡

Week of: _____

Goals for the Week:

Monday

Tuesday

Wednesday

← Clip for current week

Notes:

Thursday

Friday

Saturday/Sunday

Clip for current week ➤

Week of: _____

Goals for the Week:

Monday

Tuesday

Wednesday

← Clip for current week

Notes:

Thursday

Friday

Saturday/Sunday

Planner—Weekly

Clip for current week ➡

Week of: _____

Goals for the Week:

Monday

Tuesday

Wednesday

← Clip for current week

Notes:

Thursday

Friday

Saturday/Sunday

Clip for current week ➡

Week of: _____

Goals for the Week:

Monday

Tuesday

Wednesday

← Clip for current week

Notes:

Thursday

Friday

Saturday/Sunday

Clip for current week ➡

Week of: _____

Goals for the Week:

Monday

Tuesday

Wednesday

← Clip for current week

Notes:

Thursday

Friday

Saturday/Sunday

Clip for current week ➡

RESUME BUILDER
TEMPLATE FORM
*Contents in italics are for your reference only
and should not be included in the final resume.*

Name
Address
Phone
Email

Objective: *(What job you are seeking and why, a sentence or two)* _____

Experience:
Take 3–4 from the Resume Builder—Experience List in this section. Choose the ones most applicable to the job for which you are applying. (Use the stories in the interview, not on the resume.)

From: ___ *to* ___   *(Role or Job)* _____
What you did: _____
_____
_____

From: ___ *to* ___   *(Role or Job)* _____
What you did: _____
_____
_____

From: ___ *to* ___   *(Role or Job)* _____
What you did: _____
_____
_____

Education:
List in order of most relevant to job, then most recent first. List year, then degree, followed by school and city. For example: 2001   Medical Assisting Program   AA AnyCollege   Somewhere, SC

Certifications/ Licenses: *if applicable, see form in this section*
Honors/ Awards: *if applicable, see form in this section*
Activities: *if applicable, see form in this section*
Community Service/Volunteer: *if applicable, see form in this section*

References: *Upon request, see the form in this section to keep track of your references.*

NOTES

TEMPLATE FORM

Contents in italics are for your reference only
and should not be included in the final resume.

Name
Address
Phone
Email

Objective: *(What job you are seeking and why, a sentence or two)* _____

Experience:
Take 3–4 from the Resume Builder—Experience List in this section. Choose the ones most applicable to the job for which you are applying. (Use the stories in the interview, not on the resume.)

From: ___ **to** ___   **(Role or Job)** _____
What you did: _____
_____
_____

From: ___ **to** ___   **(Role or Job)** _____
What you did: _____
_____
_____

From: ___ **to** ___   **(Role or Job)** _____
What you did: _____
_____
_____

Education:
List in order of most relevant to job, then most recent first. List year, then degree, followed by school and city. For example: 2001   Medical Assisting Program   AA AnyCollege   Somewhere, SC

Certifications/ Licenses: *if applicable, see form in this section*
Honors/ Awards: *if applicable, see form in this section*
Activities: *if applicable, see form in this section*
Community Service/Volunteer: *if applicable, see form in this section*

References: *Upon request, see the form in this section to keep track of your references.*

NOTES

RESUME BUILDER
TEMPLATE FORM
*Contents in italics are for your reference only
and should not be included in the final resume.*

Name
Address
Phone
Email

Objective: *(What job you are seeking and why, a sentence or two)* _____

Experience:
Take 3–4 from the Resume Builder—Experience List in this section. Choose the ones most applicable to the job for which you are applying. (Use the stories in the interview, not on the resume.)

From: ____ *to* ____   *(Role or Job)* _____
What you did: _____
_____
_____

From: ____ *to* ____   *(Role or Job)* _____
What you did: _____
_____
_____

From: ____ *to* ____   *(Role or Job)* _____
What you did: _____
_____
_____

Education:
List in order of most relevant to job, then most recent first. List year, then degree, followed by school and city. For example: 2001   Medical Assisting Program   AA AnyCollege   Somewhere, SC

Certifications/ Licenses: *if applicable, see form in this section*
Honors/ Awards: *if applicable, see form in this section*
Activities: *if applicable, see form in this section*
Community Service/Volunteer: *if applicable, see form in this section*

References: *Upon request, see the form in this section to keep track of your references.*

RESUME BUILDER
NOTES

RESUME BUILDER
SKILLS AND KNOWLEDGE FORM

Skill or Knowledge	When	Experience/Application	Proof/Notes

Career Planning

RESUME BUILDER
SKILLS AND KNOWLEDGE FORM

Skill or Knowledge	When	Experience/Application	Proof/Notes

Career Planning

RESUME BUILDER

SKILLS AND KNOWLEDGE FORM

Skill or Knowledge	When	Experience/Application	Proof/Notes

Career Planning

RESUME BUILDER

SKILLS AND KNOWLEDGE FORM

Skill or Knowledge	When	Experience/Application	Proof/Notes

SKILLS AND KNOWLEDGE FORM

Skill or Knowledge	When	Experience/Application	Proof/Notes

Career Planning

Career Planning

RESUME BUILDER
SKILLS AND KNOWLEDGE FORM

Skill or Knowledge	When	Experience/Application	Proof/Notes

RESUME BUILDER

EXPERIENCES FORM

Experiences: (Clinical, job, externship, etc)

From _____ to _____   Supervisor: _____ phone: _____

What was your role or position? _____

What did you do (use your skills list from this section, also use active resume verbs from this section)?

_____

_____

_____

_____

_____

_____

_____

_____

_____

Story: Give an example of your leadership, your initiative, your caring or any other positive trait. Work these stories in during your interview.

_____

_____

_____

_____

_____

_____

_____

_____

_____

_____

_____

Career Planning

RESUME BUILDER
EXPERIENCES FORM

Experiences: (Clinical, job, externship, etc)

From _____ to _____   Supervisor: _____   phone: _____

What was your role or position? _____

What did you do (use your skills list from this section, also use active resume verbs from this section)?

_____

_____

_____

_____

_____

_____

_____

_____

Career Planning

Story: Give an example of your leadership, your initiative, your caring or any other positive trait. Work these stories in during your interview.

_____

_____

_____

_____

_____

_____

_____

_____

_____

RESUME BUILDER
EXPERIENCES FORM

Experiences: (Clinical, job, externship, etc)

From _____ to _____   Supervisor: _____   phone: _____

What was your role or position? _____

What did you do (use your skills list from this section, also use active resume verbs from this section)?

_____

_____

_____

_____

_____

_____

_____

_____

_____

Story: Give an example of your leadership, your initiative, your caring or any other positive trait. Work these stories in during your interview.

_____

_____

_____

_____

_____

_____

_____

_____

_____

_____

_____

_____

Career Planning

EXPERIENCES FORM

Experiences: (Clinical, job, externship, etc)

From _____ to _____   Supervisor: _____   phone: _____

What was your role or position? _____

What did you do (use your skills list from this section, also use active resume verbs from this section)?

_____

_____

_____

_____

_____

_____

_____

_____

_____

Story: Give an example of your leadership, your initiative, your caring or any other positive trait. Work these stories in during your interview.

_____

_____

_____

_____

_____

_____

_____

_____

_____

_____

_____

Career Planning

RESUME BUILDER
EXPERIENCES FORM

Experiences: (Clinical, job, externship, etc)

From _____ to _____   Supervisor: _____ phone: _____

What was your role or position? _____

What did you do (use your skills list from this section, also use active resume verbs from this section)?

_____

_____

_____

_____

_____

_____

_____

_____

_____

Story: Give an example of your leadership, your initiative, your caring or any other positive trait. Work these stories in during your interview.

_____

_____

_____

_____

_____

_____

_____

_____

_____

_____

Career Planning

RESUME BUILDER
EXPERIENCES FORM

Experiences: (Clinical, job, externship, etc)

From _____ to _____   Supervisor: _____   phone: _____

What was your role or position? _____

What did you do (use your skills list from this section, also use active resume verbs from this section)?

_____

_____

_____

_____

_____

_____

_____

_____

_____

Story: Give an example of your leadership, your initiative, your caring or any other positive trait. Work these stories in during your interview.

_____

_____

_____

_____

_____

_____

_____

_____

_____

_____

_____

Career Planning

RESUME BUILDER
EXPERIENCES FORM

Experiences: (Clinical, job, externship, etc)

From _____ to _____   Supervisor: _____ phone: _____

What was your role or position? _____

What did you do (use your skills list from this section, also use active resume verbs from this section)?

_____

_____

_____

_____

_____

_____

_____

_____

_____

Story: Give an example of your leadership, your initiative, your caring or any other positive trait. Work these stories in during your interview.

_____

_____

_____

_____

_____

_____

_____

_____

_____

_____

Career Planning

EXPERIENCES FORM

Experiences: (Clinical, job, externship, etc)

From _____ to _____   Supervisor: _____   phone: _____

What was your role or position? _____

What did you do (use your skills list from this section, also use active resume verbs from this section)?

_____

_____

_____

_____

_____

_____

_____

_____

_____

Story: Give an example of your leadership, your initiative, your caring or any other positive trait. Work these stories in during your interview.

_____

_____

_____

_____

_____

_____

_____

_____

_____

_____

_____

_____

Career Planning

EXPERIENCES FORM

Experiences: (Clinical, job, externship, etc)

From _____ to _____   Supervisor: _____ phone: _____

What was your role or position? _____

What did you do (use your skills list from this section, also use active resume verbs from this section)?

_____

_____

_____

_____

_____

_____

_____

_____

_____

Story: Give an example of your leadership, your initiative, your caring or any other positive trait. Work these stories in during your interview.

_____

_____

_____

_____

_____

_____

_____

_____

_____

_____

_____

Career Planning

EXPERIENCES FORM

Experiences: (Clinical, job, externship, etc)

From _____ to _____   Supervisor: _____   phone: _____

What was your role or position? _____

What did you do (use your skills list from this section, also use active resume verbs from this section)?

_____

_____

_____

_____

_____

_____

_____

_____

_____

Story: Give an example of your leadership, your initiative, your caring or any other positive trait. Work these stories in during your interview.

_____

_____

_____

_____

_____

_____

_____

_____

_____

_____

_____

Career Planning

RESUME BUILDER
ACTIVITIES FORM

Activity	Organization	Date	Notes

Career Planning

RESUME BUILDER
ACTIVITIES FORM

Activity	Organization	Date	Notes

RESUME BUILDER
ACTIVITIES FORM

Activity	Organization	Date	Notes

Career Planning

RESUME BUILDER
ACTIVITIES FORM

Activity	Organization	Date	Notes

Career Planning

LICENSES/CERTIFICATIONS FORM

License or Certification	Date	Organization	Renewal Information	Notes

Career Planning

RESUME BUILDER
LICENSES/CERTIFICATIONS FORM

License or Certification	Date	Organization	Renewal Information	Notes

LICENSES/CERTIFICATIONS FORM

License or Certification	Date	Organization	Renewal Information	Notes

Career Planning

LICENSES/CERTIFICATIONS FORM

License or Certification	Date	Organization	Renewal Information	Notes

RESUME BUILDER
AWARDS AND HONORS FORM

Award/Honor	From (Organization)	Date	Explanation/Story

Career Planning

RESUME BUILDER
AWARDS AND HONORS FORM

Award/Honor	From (Organization)	Date	Explanation/Story

COMMUNITY SERVICE & VOLUNTEER WORK FORM

What/Where	Date(s)	Organization	Contact Person/ Phone	Notes

Career Planning

RESUME BUILDER

COMMUNITY SERVICE & VOLUNTEER WORK FORM

What/Where	Date(s)	Organization	Contact Person/ Phone	Notes

Career Planning

RESUME BUILDER
COMMUNITY SERVICE & VOLUNTEER WORK FORM

What/Where	Date(s)	Organization	Contact Person/ Phone	Notes

Career Planning

RESUME BUILDER

COMMUNITY SERVICE & VOLUNTEER WORK FORM

What/Where	Date(s)	Organization	Contact Person/ Phone	Notes

RESUME BUILDER

COMMUNITY SERVICE &
VOLUNTEER WORK FORM

What/Where	Date(s)	Organization	Contact Person/ Phone	Notes

RESUME BUILDER
REFERENCES FORM

Name	Address	Phone	OK to use?	For What Job or Trait?

Career Planning

RESUME BUILDER
REFERENCES FORM

Name	Address	Phone	OK to use?	For What Job or Trait?

Career Planning

RESUME BUILDER
REFERENCES FORM

Name	Address	Phone	OK to use?	For What Job or Trait?

Career Planning

RESUME BUILDER

REFERENCES FORM

Name	Address	Phone	OK to use?	For What Job or Trait?

Career Planning

RESUME BUILDER
REFERENCES FORM

Name	Address	Phone	OK to use?	For What Job or Trait?

Active Verbs for Use on Resumes

Achieved	Handled	Performed
Administered	Helped	Planned
Assisted	Hired	Prepared
Billed	Implemented	Presented
Budgeted	Improved	Produced
Calculated	Increased	Provided
Cared for	Influenced	Purchased
Coded	Informed	Recorded
Communicated	Initiated	Regulated
Composed	Inspired	Repaired
Constructed	Instructed	Reported
Controlled	Introduced	Represented
Coordinated	Justified	Revised
Created	Launched	Scheduled
Demonstrated	Led	Secured
Designed	Maintained	Set up
Developed	Managed	Showed
Directed	Monitored	Sold
Documented	Motivated	Supervised
Educated	Negotiated	Taught
Encouraged	Obtained	Tested
Established	Operated	Trained
Expanded	Ordered	Verified
Generated	Organized	Word processed
Greeted	Participated	Wrote

From: Haroun, L. (2000). Career Development for Health Professionals. Phila.: W B Saunders, p.208, Box 9-1. Reprinted with permission.

Career Planning

Resume Checklist

_____   Dates and numbers are complete and accurate.

_____   Your phone number is included.

_____   The objective is clear.

_____   Content supports the objective.

_____   Content is organized in order of importance.

_____   All important qualifications are included.

_____   Information is not repeated.

_____   Spelling is perfect.

_____   Grammar is correct.

_____   Layout is consistent.

_____   The page is attractively laid out.

From: Haroun, L. (2000). Career Development for Health Professionals. Phila.: W B Saunders, p. 219, Box 9-2. Reprinted with permission.

Career Planning

INTERVIEW FORM

Position: _____   Date/Time of Interview: _____

Person Interviewing: _____   Start Date: _____

His/her position: _____   Salary (Range): _____

Phone Number: _____   Benefits: Y   N

Place of Interview and Directions: _____

_____

_____

NOTES:

_____

_____

_____

_____

Steps to a Great Interview
Remember You are a great "product"!
List 3 strong features you have that fit this job opportunity:

1. _____

2. _____

3. _____

Bring at least two copies of your resume.

Arrive at least 15 minutes early for the interview.

Tell your stories from the Resume Builder Experience Form in this section. These examples or stories should be less than 2 minutes each practice them! Stories/Examples for this interview:

_____

_____

_____

_____

Be enthusiastic and interested in the company and industry.
Learn a bit about the company before the interview if you can.
Notes about the company:

_____

_____

_____

Make eye contact. Smile. Listen actively and respond confidently.

Ask questions. Brainstorm a few questions in the space below.

_____

_____

_____

Ask what happens next in the process. Note the next step in the space below:

_____

_____

Thank him, her, or them for the interview.

Follow Up:

1. Thank You Note sent (who and when):

   _____

2. Follow Up Call:

   _____

3. 2nd Follow Up:

   _____

4. What happened:

   _____

   _____

What I liked about this job opportunity:

_____

_____

What I did well:

_____

_____

Things to do differently next time:

_____

_____

Other Thoughts/Notes:

_____

_____

_____

_____

_____

Career Planning

INTERVIEW FORM

Position: _____   Date/Time of Interview: _____

Person Interviewing: _____   Start Date: _____

His/her position: _____   Salary (Range): _____

Phone Number: _____   Benefits: Y   N

Place of Interview and Directions: _____

_____

_____

NOTES:

_____

_____

_____

_____

Steps to a Great Interview
Remember You are a great "product"!
    List 3 strong features you have that fit this job opportunity:

     1. _____

     2. _____

     3. _____

Bring at least two copies of your resume.

Arrive at least 15 minutes early for the interview.

**Tell your stories from the Resume Builder Experience Form
in this section.** These examples or stories should be less than 2
minutes each practice them! Stories/Examples for this interview:

_____

_____

_____

_____

Be enthusiastic and interested in the company and industry.
Learn a bit about the company before the interview if you can.
Notes about the company:

_____

_____

_____

**Make eye contact. Smile. Listen actively and respond
confidently.**

Ask questions. Brainstorm a few questions in the space below.

_____
_____
_____

Ask what happens next in the process. Note the next step in the
space below:

_____
_____

Thank him, her, or them for the interview.

Follow Up:

   1. Thank You Note sent (who and when):

      _____

   2. Follow Up Call:

      _____

   3. 2nd Follow Up:

      _____

   4. What happened:

      _____
      _____

What I liked about this job opportunity:

_____
_____

What I did well:

_____
_____

Things to do differently next time:

_____
_____

Other Thoughts/Notes:

_____
_____
_____
_____
_____

Career Planning

INTERVIEW FORM

Position: _____ Date/Time of Interview: _____
Person Interviewing: _____ Start Date: _____
  His/her position: _____ Salary (Range): _____
Phone Number: _____ Benefits: Y   N

Place of Interview and Directions: _____
_____
_____

NOTES:
_____
_____
_____
_____

Steps to a Great Interview
Remember You are a great "product"!
   List 3 strong features you have that fit this job opportunity:
    1. _____
    2. _____
    3. _____

Bring at least two copies of your resume.

Arrive at least 15 minutes early for the interview.

Tell your stories from the Resume Builder Experience Form in this section. These examples or stories should be less than 2 minutes each practice them! Stories/Examples for this interview:
_____
_____
_____
_____

Be enthusiastic and interested in the company and industry.
Learn a bit about the company before the interview if you can. Notes about the company:
_____
_____
_____

Make eye contact. Smile. Listen actively and respond confidently.

Ask questions. Brainstorm a few questions in the space below.

_____

_____

_____

Ask what happens next in the process. Note the next step in the space below:

_____

_____

Thank him, her, or them for the interview.

Follow Up:

1. Thank You Note sent (who and when):

   _____

2. Follow Up Call:

   _____

3. 2nd Follow Up:

   _____

4. What happened:

   _____

   _____

What I liked about this job opportunity:

   _____

   _____

What I did well:

   _____

   _____

Things to do differently next time:

   _____

   _____

Other Thoughts/Notes:

_____

_____

_____

_____

_____

_____

Career Planning

INTERVIEW FORM

Position: _____   Date/Time of Interview: _____

Person Interviewing: _____   Start Date: _____

   His/her position: _____   Salary (Range): _____

Phone Number: _____   Benefits: Y   N

Place of Interview and Directions: _____

_____

_____

NOTES:

_____

_____

_____

_____

Steps to a Great Interview

Remember You are a great "product"!

List 3 strong features you have that fit this job opportunity:

1. _____

2. _____

3. _____

Bring at least two copies of your resume.

Arrive at least 15 minutes early for the interview.

Tell your stories from the Resume Builder Experience Form in this section. These examples or stories should be less than 2 minutes each practice them! Stories/Examples for this interview:

_____

_____

_____

_____

Be enthusiastic and interested in the company and industry.

Learn a bit about the company before the interview if you can. Notes about the company:

_____

_____

_____

Make eye contact. Smile. Listen actively and respond confidently.

Ask questions. Brainstorm a few questions in the space below.

_____

_____

_____

Ask what happens next in the process. Note the next step in the space below:

_____

_____

Thank him, her, or them for the interview.

Follow Up:

1. Thank You Note sent (who and when):

   _____

2. Follow Up Call:

   _____

3. 2nd Follow Up:

   _____

4. What happened:

   _____

   _____

What I liked about this job opportunity:

_____

_____

What I did well:

_____

_____

Things to do differently next time:

_____

_____

Other Thoughts/Notes:

_____

_____

_____

_____

_____

_____

INTERVIEW FORM

Position: _____ Date/Time of Interview: _____

Person Interviewing: _____ Start Date: _____

His/her position: _____ Salary (Range): _____

Phone Number: _____ Benefits: Y   N

Place of Interview and Directions: _____

_____

_____

NOTES:

_____

_____

_____

_____

Steps to a Great Interview

Remember You are a great "product"!

   List 3 strong features you have that fit this job opportunity:

   1. _____

   2. _____

   3. _____

Bring at least two copies of your resume.

Arrive at least 15 minutes early for the interview.

Tell your stories from the Resume Builder Experience Form in this section. These examples or stories should be less than 2 minutes each practice them! Stories/Examples for this interview:

_____

_____

_____

_____

Be enthusiastic and interested in the company and industry.
Learn a bit about the company before the interview if you can. Notes about the company:

_____

_____

_____

Make eye contact. Smile. Listen actively and respond confidently.

Ask questions. Brainstorm a few questions in the space below.

_____
_____
_____

Ask what happens next in the process. Note the next step in the space below:

_____
_____

Thank him, her, or them for the interview.

Follow Up:

1. Thank You Note sent (who and when):
_____

2. Follow Up Call:
_____

3. 2nd Follow Up:
_____

4. What happened:
_____
_____

What I liked about this job opportunity:
_____
_____

What I did well:
_____
_____

Things to do differently next time:
_____
_____

Other Thoughts/Notes:

_____
_____
_____
_____
_____
_____

Professional Organizations for Health Care Occupations

Occupation	Organization	Contact Information
Cardiovascular Technologist	Alliance of Cardiovascular Professionals	910 Charles Street Fredericksburg, VA 22401
Dental Assistant	American Dental Assistants' Association	666 N. Lake Shore Drive Suite 1130 Chicago, IL 60611
Dental Hygienist	American Dental Hygienists' Association	444 N. Michigan Avenue Suite 3400 Chicago, IL 60611 www.adha.org
Dental Laboratory Technician	National Association of Dental Laboratories	8201 Greensboro Drive Suite 300 McLean, VA 22102 www.nadl.org
Diagnostic Medical Sonographer	Society of Diagnostic Medical Sonographers	12770 Coit Road Suite 708 Dallas, TX 75251

Continued

Emergency Medical Technician	National Association of Emergency Medical Technicians	408 Monroe Street Clinton, MS 39056 www.naemt.org
Health Information Technician	American Health Information Management Association	919 N. Michigan Avenue Suite 1400 Chicago, IL 60611 www.ahima.org
Medical Assistant	American Association of Medical Assistants	20 N. Wacker Drive Suite 1575 Chicago, IL 60606 www.aama-ntl.org
	American Medical Technologists' Association	710 Higgins Road Park Ridge, IL 60068 www.amt1.com
Medical Insurance Coder	American Academy of Procedural Coders	309 West 700 South Salt Lake City, UT 84101 www.aapcnatl.org
	American Health Information Management	919 N. Michigan Avenue Suite 1400 Chicago, IL 60611 www.ahima.org

Continued

Medical Laboratory Assistant/Medical Laboratory Technician	American Medical Technologists' Association	710 Higgins Road Park Ridge, IL 60068 www.amt1.com
	American Society for Clinical Laboratory Science	7910 Woodmont Avenue Suite 530 Bethesda, MD 20814 www.ascls.org
Medical Transcriptionist	American Association for Medical Transcription	3460 Oakdale Road Suite M Modesto, CA 95355 www.aamt.org
Occupational Therapy Assistant	American Occupational Therapy Association	4720 Montgomery Lane PO Box 31220 Bethesda, MD 20824 www.aota.org
Ophthalmic Laboratory Technician	Commission on Opticianry Accreditation	7023 Little River Turnpike Suite 207 Annandale, VA 22003 www.coaccreditation.com

Continued

Ophthalmic Medical Assistant	Association of Technical Personnel in Ophthalmology	PO Box 25036 St. Paul, MN 55125 www.atpo.com
Pharmacy Assistant/Technician	American Pharmaceutical Association	2215 Constitution Avenue NW Washington, DC 20037 www.aphanet.org
Phlebotomist	American Medical Technologists' Association	710 Higgins Road Park Ridge, IL 60068 www.amt1.com
Physical Therapist Assistant	American Physical Therapy Association	1111 North Fairfax Street Alexandria, VA 22314 www.apta.org
Physician Assistant	American Academy of Physician Assistants	950 N. Washington Street Alexandria, VA 22314 www.aapa.org
Practical/Vocational Nurse	National Association for Practical Nurse Education and Service, Inc.	1400 Spring Street Suite 330 Silver Springs, MD 20910 www.aoa.dhhs.gov/aoa/dir/130.html

Continued

Psychiatric/Mental Health Technician	American Association of Psychiatric Technicians	336 Johnson Road Suite 2 Michigan City, IN 46360
Radiographer/Radiologic Technologist	American Society of Radiologic Technologists	15000 Central Avenue SE Albuquerque, NM 87123 www.asrt.org
Registered Nurse	National League for Nursing	350 Hudson Street New York, NY 10014 www.nln.org
	American Nurses' Association	600 Maryland Avenue SW Suite 100 West Washington, DC 20024 www.ana.org
Respiratory Therapist	American Association for Respiratory Care	11030 Ables Lane Dallas, TX 75229 www.aarc.org
Surgical Technologist	Association of Surgical Technologists	7108-C S. Alton Way Englewood, CO 80112 www.ast.org

Directory

From: Haroun, L. (2000). Career Development for Health Professionals Phila.: W B Saunders, p. 311-313, Appendix Reprinted with permission.

Sources for Patient Education Materials and Support

Patient Education is a serious responsibility for health care professionals. Many health care facilities develop their own patient teaching materials. There are also groups, associations, businesses, and agencies that develop patient education materials for dissemination to the public. There are many tools that can be used to improve an individual's knowledge about a particular health care problem or issue. These include, but are not limited to, pamphlets, movies, videotapes, audiotapes, newsletters, and computerized instruction. Information can also be supplied to the health care professional to develop materials. The names and addresses identified below are potential sources of information that have provided information for the Miller-Keane Encyclopedia and Dictionary of Medicine, Nursing, and Allied Health. Local chapters of national organizations may also be found in the telephone directory and may serve as valuable resources for patient education material. Encyclopedias and directories of health related associations are an additional source of information on contacts.

Alcoholics Anonymous
   PO Box 49
   Grand Central Station
   New York, NY 10163
Phone: 212-870-3400
FAX: 212-870-3003
Alcoholics Anonymous is a fellowship of sober alcoholics, no dues or fees, self-supporting, no outside funds, unaffiliated; primary purpose: carry the A.A. message to alcoholic who still suffers.

Alzheimer's Disease Education and Referral Center
   PO Box 8250
   Silver Spring, MD 20907-8250
   Phone: 800-438-4380
   FAX: 301-495-3334
Provides information about Alzheimer's disease, its symptoms and diagnosis, and about Alzheimer's disease

Continued

Directory

research supported by the National Institute on Aging. Offers a newsletter to health professionals and other, free publications to the public.

Alzheimer Society of Canada
    1320 Yonge Street, Suite 201
    Toronto, Ontario M4T 1XZ
    Phone: 800-616-8816
    FAX: 416-925-3552
A national voluntary organization whose goals are to provide information and support to those affected by Alzheimer Disease and their families, to increase public awareness of Alzheimer Disease, and to search for a cause and a cure.

American Council of the Blind
    1155 15th Street NW
    Suite 720
    Washington, DC 20005
    Phone: 202-467-5081
    FAX: 202-467-5085
The American Council of the Blind is a national membership organization established to promote independence, dignity, and well-being of blind and visually impaired people. Services provided include a monthly magazine, the Braille Forum, subscriptions to which are available free of charge to individuals in the US in Braille, large print, cassettes, and 3.5 DOS diskettes, and many other services.

American Dietetic Association
    216 West Jackson Blvd.
    Chicago, IL 60606
    Phone: 312-899-0040
    Toll Free: 800-366-1655 (Consumer Hot Line)
The American Dietetic Association (ADA) promotes the optimal health, nutrition, and well-being of the public. The National Center for Nutrition and Dietetics maintains a consumer nutrition hotline that provides information and referrals to registered dietitians throughout the country.

Directory

Continued

The Amyotrophic Lateral Sclerosis Association
21021 Ventura Boulevard, Suite 321
Woodland Hills, CA 91364-2206
Phone: 818-340-7500
FAX: 818-340-2060
Toll Free: 800-782-4747
The mission of the ALS Association is to discover the cause
and cure for amyotrophic lateral sclerosis (Lou Gehrig's
disease) through dedicated research while providing patient
support, information/education for health care professionals
and the general public, and advocacy for ALS research and
health care concerns.

Association of Community Cancer Centers
11600 Nebel Street, Suite 201
Rockville, MD 20852
Phone: 301-984-9496
The mission of the Association of Community Cancer
Centers is to promote the continuum of quality cancer care
(research, prevention, screening, early detection, diagnosis,
treatment, psychosocial services, rehabilitation, hospice)
for patients with cancer and the community.

Asthma and Allergy Foundation of America (AAFA)
1125 15th Street, NW, Suite 502
Washington, DC 20005
Phone: 202-466-7943
FAX: 202-466-8940
AAFA has been in existence for over forty years and is a
registered not-for-profit patient education organization
dedicated to finding a cure for and controlling asthma and
allergic diseases.

Bulimia Anorexia Nervosa Association (BANA)
3640 Wells Avenue
Windsor, Ontario N9C 1T9
Phone: 519-253-7545
The objectives of BANA are to eradicate eating disorders;
to promote healthy eating and acceptance of diverse body
shapes; and to provide clinical, preventive, and advocacy
services for persons affected by eating disorders.

Continued

Directory

Canada Safety Council

> 1020 Thomas Spratt Place
> Ottawa, Ontario K1G 5L5
> Phone: 613-739-1535

The Canada Safety Council is Canada's national not-for-profit safety organization. Its mission is to be a leader in the effort to reduce preventable deaths, injuries, and economic loss in the traffic, work, home community, and leisure environments.

Canadian Cystic Fibrosis Foundation

> 2221 Yonge Street Suite 601
> Toronto, Ontario
> Phone: 416-485-9149
> FAX: 416-485-0960

The purpose and objectives of the Canadian Cystic Fibrosis Foundation are to aid those afflicted with cystic fibrosis; to conduct research into improved care and treatment and to seek a cure or control for cystic fibrosis; to promote public awareness through the dissemination of information using all forms of communication; and to raise funds and allocate same for the above purposes.

Canadian Hard of Hearing Association

> (CHHA) 2435 Holly Lane Suite 205
> Ottawa, Ontario K1V 7P2
> Voice Phone: 613-526-1584
> FAX: 613-526-4718
> TTY: 613-526-2692
> Toll Free: 800-263-8068

The Canadian Hard of Hearing Association is the "voice" of hard of hearing Canada. CHHA is the only Canadian, national, non-profit consumer organization run by and for hard of hearing people. CHHA exists to help the hard of hearing achieve independent, productive, and fulfilling lives.

Canadian Mental Health Association—National

> 2160 Yonge Street, Third Floor
> Toronto, Ontario M4S 2Z3
> Phone: 416-484-7750
> FAX: 416-484-4617

Directory

Continued

The Canadian Mental Health Association is a national voluntary association that exists to promote the mental health of all people. CMHA's mission is operationalized through education, advocacy, research, service provision, and facilitation.

Canadian National Institute for the Blind (CNIB)
1929 Bayview Avenue
Toronto, Ontario M4G 3E8
Phone: 416-486-2500

CNIB is the world's largest provider of services to people with visual impairments, and a global leader in adaptive and assistive technologies.

Cancer Care, Inc.
1180 Avenue of the Americas
New York, NY 10036
Phone: 800-813-HOPE

Offers information, referral, individual and group counseling, and patient education free of charge.

Centers for Disease Control and Prevention (CDC)
1600 Clifton Road, NE
Atlanta, GA 30333

Provides information on diseases, health risks, prevention guidelines, and strategies. A wide variety of services can be accessed through the CDC.

Clinical Reference Systems, Ltd.
7100 E. Belleview Avenue, Suite 208
Greenwood Village, CO 80111-1636
Phone: 800-237-8401
FAX: 303-220-1685
Contact: Sales Department

Software designed to generate patient education handouts on IBM and compatible PCs in a wide variety of areas. Editing of topics and customizing of handouts is a feature.

Continued

Directory

Crohn's and Colitis Foundation of Canada (CCFC)

301-21 St. Clair Avenue E.
Toronto, Ontario M4T 1L9
Phone: 416-920-5035
FAX: 416-929-0364
Toll Free: 800-387-1479 (Canada only)

The Crohn's and Colitis Foundation of Canada (CCFC) is a national not-for-profit voluntary Foundation dedicated to finding the cure for Crohn's disease and ulcerative colitis. To realize this the Foundation is committed to raise increasing funds for research. The CCFC also believes that it is important to make all individuals with inflammatory bowel disease aware of the Foundation, and to educate these individuals, their families, health professionals, and the general public.

Cystic Fibrosis Foundation

6931 Arlington Road
Bethesda, MD 20814
Phone: 301-951-4422
FAX: 301-951-6378
Toll Free: 800-344-4823

The Cystic Fibrosis Foundation was established in 1955 to raise money to fund research to find a cure for cystic fibrosis and to improve the quality of life for the 30,000 children and young adults with the disease.

Endometriosis Association International Headquarters

8585 N. 76th Place
Milwaukee, WI 53223
Phone: 414-355-2200
FAX: 414-355-6065
Toll Free: 800-992-3636

The Endometriosis Association is a self-help organization dedicated to offering support and information to women with Endometriosis, educating the public and medical community about the disease, and promoting and conducting research related to Endometriosis.

Directory

Continued

The Epilepsy Foundation of America

4321 Garden City Drive
Landover, MD 20785
Phone: 301-459-3700
Toll Free: 800-EFA-1000

The Epilepsy Foundation of America is the national organization that works for people affected by seizures, through research, education, advocacy, and service.

International Federation on Aging (IFA)

380 Rue Saint-Antoine Quest
Bureau 3200
Montreal, Quebec H2Y 3X7
Phone: 514-287-9679

IFA serves as an advocate for the well-being of older persons around the world. IFA is committed to providing a worldwide forum on aging issues and concerns and to fostering the development of associations and agencies that serve or represent older persons.

La Leche League Canada

Box 29 18C Industrial Drive
Chesterville, Ontario KOC 1HO
Phone: 613-448-1842
FAX: 613-448-1845

La Leche League Canada promotes a better understanding of breastfeeding as an important element in the healthy development of the baby, and through education, information, encouragement, and mother-to-mother support helps mothers nationwide to breastfeed. The main objective of La Leche League Canada is to help mothers breastfeed their babies.

Learning Disabilities Association of America

4156 Library Road
Pittsburgh, PA 15234
Phone: 412-341-1515

LDA is an information and referral organization. We provide any and all information regarding learning disabilities in both children and adults. There are 500 chapters across the country. Once individuals make contact with us, we provide a free packet of material, then refer them on to one of our chapters. We also offer membership.

Continued

National Asian Pacific Center on Aging
Melbourne Tower, Suite 914
1511 Third Avenue
Seattle, WA 98101-1626
Phone: 206-624-1221
FAX: 206-624-1023

The National Asian Pacific Center on Aging (NAPCA) is the leading advocacy organization committed to the well-being of elderly Asians and Pacific Islanders in America. NAPCA develops and administers programs to enhance the dignity and quality of life of its constituents. NAPCA provides a fax-on-demand service for over 300 pamphlets, brochures, fact sheets, etc. in 15 languages on topics related to health, wellness, social services, and related topics. FAX-IT can be reached by dialing 206-624-0185 from any FAX machine (telephone handset).

National Association for Medical Equipment Services (NAHMES)
625 Slaters Lane, Suite 200
Alexandria, VA 22314-1171
Phone: 703-836-6263
FAX: 703-836-6730

The National Association for Medical Equipment Services (NAHMES) is headquartered in Alexandria, VA. Formed in 1982, it is the only national association representing the home health medical equipment (HME) services industry exclusively. NAHMES' mission is to promote access to quality HME services and rehabilitation/assistive technology as an integral part of our nation's health care system.

National Association for Visually Handicapped
22 West 21st Street
New York, NY 10010
Phone: 212-889-3134

To promote hope, dignity, and productivity for those with uncorrectable visual impairments by encouraging the full use of residual vision through large print, visual aids, emotional support, educational outreach, advocacy, and referral services.

Directory

Continued

National Cancer Institute Information Associates Program

> 9300 Old Georgetown Road
> Bethesda, MD 20814-1519
> Phone: 301-496-7600
> Toll Free: 800-624-7890

Provides access to the National Cancer Institute's information resources for health professionals, including the journal of the National Cancer Institute.

National Clearinghouse for Alcohol and Drug Information (NCADI)

> 11426 Rockville Pike, Suite 200
> Rockville, MD 20852-3007
> Phone: 800-729-6686
> TDD: 800-487-4889
> FAX: 301-468-6433

A service of the U.S. Center for Substance Abuse Prevention, NCADI collects and distributes information about alcohol, tobacco, and other drugs to all interested persons. The Clearinghouse provides a wide variety of free printed material; also videotapes and disk-based products for a small cost-recovery fee.

National Clearinghouse on Child Abuse and Neglect Information

> PO Box 1182
> Washington, DC 20013-1182
> Phone: 800-394-3366

The Clearinghouse collects, catalogues, stores, organizes, and disseminates information on all aspects of child maltreatment.

National Committee for the Prevention of Elder Abuse

> c/o Institute on Aging
> The Medical Center of Central Massachusetts
> 119 Belmont Street
> Worcester, MA 01605

The National Committee for the Prevention of Elder Abuse was established to promote greater understanding of elder abuse and the development of services to protect older persons and disabled adults and reduce the likelihood of their being abused, neglected, and/or exploited.

Continued

National Council on Alcoholism and Drug Dependence, Inc.
12 West 21st St.
New York, NY 10010
Phone: 800-NCA-Call

The National Council on Alcoholism and Drug Dependence, Inc. provides education, information, help, and hope in the fight against the chronic and often fatal disease of alcoholism, and other drug addictions. Founded in 1944, NCADD, with its nationwide network of affiliates, advocates prevention, intervention, and treatment, and is committed to ridding the disease of its stigma and its sufferers of their denial and shame.

National Health Council
1730 M Street, NW, Suite 500
Washington, DC 20036
Phone: 202-785-3910

The National Health Council is a private, nonprofit association of national organizations which was founded in 1920 as a clearinghouse and cooperative effort for voluntary health agencies (VHAs).

The National Institute of Nutrition (NIN)
265 Carling Avenue, Suite 302
Ottawa, Ontario K1S 2E1
Phone: 613-235-3355

Founded in 1983, NIN is a private, nonprofit national organization dedicated to bridging the gap between the science and practice of nutrition and serving as a credible source of information on nutrition. The NIN also conducts and supports nutrition research.

National Wellness Institute
1045 Clark Street, Suite 210
P.O. Box 827
Stevens Point, WI 54481-0827
Phone: 715-342-2969

The National Wellness Institute has served professionals interested in wellness and health promotion since 1977. It focuses on professional education programs; resources and information dissemination through its professional association, the National Wellness Association; and the development and distribution of lifestyle inventories and health risk appraisals.

Directory

Continued

The Nemours Foundation
> The Alfred I. duPont Institute
> 1600 Rockland Road
> Wilmington, DE 19803

Maintains a very informative site on the world wide web known as Kidshealth.

Osteoporosis Society of Canada
> 33 Laird Drive
> Toronto, Ontario M5S 3A7
> Phone: 416-696-2817
> Toll Free (Canada only): 800-463-6842

To educate and empower individuals and communities in the prevention and treatment of osteoporosis. We are a resource for patients, health professionals, the media, and the general public who seek medically accurate information on the causes, prevention, and treatment of osteoporosis.

Pregnancy and Infant Loss Center
> 1421 East Wayzata Boulevard #30
> Wayzata, MN 55391
> Phone: 612-473-9372
> FAX: 612-473-8978

A national nonprofit organization, founded in 1983, providing support, resources, and education on miscarriage, stillbirth, and infant death.

Pregnancy & Infant Loss Support, Inc. (SHARE)
> National Office
> St. Joseph Health Center
> 300 First Capitol Drive
> St. Charles, MO 63301
> Phone: 800-821-6819
> FAX: 314-947-7486

SHARE offers support to families and caregivers whose lives have been touched by the tragic death of a baby through miscarriage, stillbirth, or newborn death by providing information, education, and a network of support groups across the country.

Continued

Directory

Recording for the Blind and Dyslexic (RFB & D)
20 Roszel Road
Princeton, NJ 08540
Phone: 609-452-0606
Toll Free: 800-221-4792

RFB & D maintains the world's largest collection of professional resources and textbooks on audio tape for all academic levels. It serves people who cannot read standard print because of a visual, perceptual, or other physical disability.

SIECUS
(Sexuality Information and Education Council of the United States)
Publication Department
130 West 42nd Street, Suite 350
New York, NY 10036-7802
Phone: 212-819-9770

SIECUS affirms that sexuality is a natural and healthy part of living. SIECUS develops, collects, and disseminates information, promotes comprehensive education about sexuality, and advocates the right of individuals to make responsible sexual choices.

Students Against Drunk Driving (SADD)
255 Main Street
PO Box 800
Marlboro, MA 01752
Phone: 508-481-3568
FAX: 508-481-5759

To provide young people with the tools to address the problems of underage drinking, impaired driving, drug use, and their consequences.

Continued

Directory

UNOS
United Network for Organ Sharing

>1100 Boulders Parkway, Suite 500
>Richmond, VA 23225
>Phone: 804-330-8500

UNOS, under contract with the U.S. Department of Health and Human Services, is a nonprofit organization that administers the National Organ Procurement and Transplantation Network (OPTN) and the U.S. Scientific Registry of Organ Transplant Recipients mandated by Congress. It operates and maintains the national list of patients waiting for solid organ transplants. In addition, it maintains a computer assisted system for allocating organs to individuals on the waiting list. The primary goal of the UNOS organization is to increase the number of donated organs. Through a number of strategies, including public and professional education, UNOS endeavors to bridge the gap between the number of individuals waiting for transplant and the number of organs donated. Information about organ donation and transplantation is available from UNOS 24 hours a day, 365 days a year.

From: Miller/Keane: Encyclopedia & Dictionary of Medicine, Nursing, & Allied Health (6th ed.). Philadelphia: WB Saunders, p.1880-1883. Reprinted with permission.

Directory

Patient Advocacy Telephone Numbers

Toll-free and other patient advocacy lines offering a variety of services to patients and health care professionals are listed below. Please verify that the number remains correct before sharing this information with patients. The Johns Hopkins School of Medicine, Division of Biomedical Information Sciences maintains a frequently updated list on the World Wide Web that can be reached at: http://infonet.welch.jhu.edu/advocacy.html

Advocacy
201-625-7101 American Self-Help Clearinghouse
800-48-FRIEND The Friends' Health Connection
407-253-9048 Med Help International

Aging
800-424-2277 American Association of Retired Persons
800-222-3937 National Eye Care Project

AIDS
800-458-5231 National AIDS Information Clearinghouse
800-342-AIDS National AIDS Hotline
800-669-0696 AIDS Education at Work
800-673-8538 National Association of People with AIDS

Alcohol
800-622-2255 National Council on Alcoholism
800-344-2666 Al-Anon, Alateen Family Group Hotline
800-527-5344 American Council on Alcoholism
800-729-6686 National Clearinghouse for Alcohol and
 Drug Information

Allergy
800-822-2762 American Academy of Allergy, Asthma &
 Immunology
800-727-8462 Asthma and Allergy Foundation of America

Alzheimer's
800-272-3900 Alzheimer's Association
800-621-0379 Alzheimer's Disease and Related Disorders
800-477-2243 French Foundation for Alzheimer's Research

Amyotrophic Lateral Sclerosis
800-782-4747 Amyotrophic Lateral Sclerosis Association

Continued

Arthritis
800-283-7800 Arthritis Foundation
800-327-3027 Arthritis Consulting Services

Ataxia
800-5-HELP-AT Ataxia Telangiectasia Children's Project
612-473-7666 National Ataxia Foundation

Back Pain
800-247-2225 Back Pain Hotline

Biliary Atresia
718-987-6200 Biliary Atresia and Liver Transplant
    Network

Birth Defects
800-221-6827 National Easter Seal Society

Blind/Vision Impaired
800-683-5555 Foundation Fighting Blindness
800-424-8666 National Alliance of Blind Students
800-232-5463 American Foundation for the Blind
800-562-6265 National Association of Parents of Visually
    Impaired
800-334-5497 National Center for Vision and Ageng
800-548-4337 Guide Dog Foundation for the Blind
800-424-8567 National Library Services for the Blind and
    Physically Handicapped

Brain Tumors
800-886-2282 American Brain Tumor Association
800-934-CURE National Brain Tumor Foundation

Cancer
510-204-4286 Alta Bates-Herrick Breast Cancer Risk
    Counseling
800-525-3777 AMC Information and Counseling Line
800-ACS-2345 American Cancer Society
800-4-CANCER Cancer Information Service
800-843-8114 American Institute for Cancer Research
301-984-9496 The Association of Community Cancer
    Centers
800-366-2223 Candelighters Childhood Cancer Foundation
800-55-CHEMO CHEMOcare
800-ICARE-61 The International Cancer Alliance, Inc.

Continued

Directory

800-452-CURE International Myeloma Foundation

212-719-0154 National Alliance of Breast Cancer
Organizations (NABCO)

202-296-7477 National Breast Cancer Coalition

800-4-CANCER National Cancer Institute

301-650-8868 National Coalition for Cancer Survivorship

301-496-7403 NCI's CancerFax

616-453-1477 Patient Advocates for Advanced Cancer
Treatment

212-719-0364 SHARE

800-IM-AWARE The Susan G. Komen Breast Cancer
Foundation

708-323-1002 US TOO International (Prostate Cancer/
BPH)

800-221-2141 Y-ME Breast Cancer Organization
(24 hrs: 312-986-8228)

Cerebral Palsy

800-872-5827 United Cerebral Palsy Association, Inc.

Children

800-433-9016 American Academy of Pediatrics

800-422-4453 Child Help USA

800-787-KIDS Children's Rights Council

800-457-6434 Human Growth Foundation (Growth
Disorders)

800-892-5437 Kidsrights

800-LA LECHE La Leche League International

800-872-5437 Missing Children Help Center

800-843-5678 National Center for Missing and Exploited
Children

800-422-4453 National Child Abuse Hotline

800-222-2000 National Council on Child Abuse and
Family Violence

800-543-7006 National Resource Center on Child Sexual
Abuse

Cleft Palate

800-242-5338 National Cleft Palate Association

Cocaine

800-262-2463 National Cocaine Hotline

800-347-8998 Cocaine Anonymous

Directory

Continued

Crohn's/Colitis
800-343-3637 Crohn's and Colitis Foundation of America

Chronic Fatigue Syndrome
800-442-3437 CFIDS

Cystic Fibrosis
800-344-4823 Cystic Fibrosis Foundation

Depression
800-826-3632 National Depressive & Manic-Depressive
    Association
800-248-4344 National Foundation for Depressive Illness
410-955-4647 Depression and Related Affective Disorders
    Association
516-829-0091 National Alliance for Research on
    Schizophrenia and Depression

Diabetes
800-338-DMED American Association of Diabetes
    Educators
800-223-1138 Juvenile Diabetes Foundation
800-232-3472 American Diabetes Foundation

Disabilities
407-880-9232 American Association of Disabled Persons
800-962-9629 National Spinal Cord Injury Association
800-526-3456 National Spinal Cord Injury Hotline
800-248-2253 National Organization on Disability
800-346-2742 National Rehabilitation Information Center
800-922-9234 National Information Clearinghouse for
    Infants with Disabilities and LifeThreatening Conditions

Disabilities and Life-Threatening Conditions
800-835-1043 Institute of Logopedics
800-344-5405 ABLEDATA
800-333-6293 National Center for Youth with Disabilities
800-426-2133 National Support Center for Persons with
    Disabilities

Disease Control
800-810-4000 Compliance Control Center

Divorce
800-733-DADS National Congress for Men and Children
800-457-6962 Mothers without Custody
800-637-7974 Parents without Partners

Continued

Down Syndrome
216-621-5858 The Baker Center
800-221-4602 National Down Syndrome Society
800-232-6372 National Down Syndrome Congress

Drug Abuse
800-729-6686 National Clearinghouse for Alcohol and
Drug Information
800-662-4357 CSAT's National Drug and Alcohol
Treatment Routing Service
800-667-7433 National Parents' Resource Institute for Drug
Education
800-258-2766 Just Say No International
800-662-HELP Drug Abuse Hotline

Endometriosis
800-992-3636 Endometriosis Association

Epilepsy
800-332-1000 Epilepsy Foundation of America
800-642-0500 Epilepsy Information Service

Head Injury
800-444-6443 National Head Injury Foundation

Headache
800-255-ACHE American Council for Headache Education
800-843-2256 National Headache Foundation
800-245-0088 New England Headache Treatment Program

Hearing/Communication Handicaps
800-424-8576 Better Hearing Institute
800-638-8255 American Speech Language Hearing
Association
800-535-3323 Deafness Research Foundation
800-521-5247 Hearing Aid Helpline

Hemolytic Uremic Syndrome
516-673-3017 Lois Joy Galler Foundation

Hemophilia
800-424-2634 National Hemophilia Foundation

Hepatitis
800-223-0179 American Liver Foundation Hepatitis
Foundation
800-891-0707 Hepatitis Foundation International *Continued*

Directory

Hereditary Hemorrhagic Telangiectasia

800-448-6389 HHT Foundation

Huntington's Disease

800-345-4372 Huntington's Disease Society

Immune Deficiency Foundation

800-296-4433 Immune Deficiency Foundation

Impotence

800-835-7667 Recovery of Male Potency
800-843-4315 Impotence Information Center
800-867-7042 Impotency Information sponsored by
  Pharmacia & Upjohn, Inc.

Incontinence

800-237-4666 Simon Foundation

Lupus

800-558-0121 Lupus Foundation
800-331-1802 American Lupus Society

Lymphedema

800-541-3259 National Lymphedema Network

Marfan Syndrome

800-8MARFAN National Marfan Foundation
905-826-3223 Canadian Marfan Association

Mental Health

800-447-4474 Mental Health InfoSource
207-799-6750 Creative Health Foundation

Mental Retardation

817-261-6003 The Arc

Myasthenia Gravis

800-541-5454 Myasthenia Gravis Foundation

Narcolepsy

800-222-6085 American Narcolepsy Association
800-829-1933 Narcolepsy & Sleep Disorders

Nutrition

800-877-1600 American Dietetic Association

Organ Transplantation

818-781-1006 American Share Foundation
800-528-2971 Living Bank International (Organ Donation)

Continued

Ostomies
800-826-0826 United Ostomy Association

Paralysis
800-225-0292 American Paralysis Association
800-962-9629 National Spinal Cord Injury Association
800-526-3456 National Spinal Cord Injury Hotline

Parkinson's Disease
800-233-2732 American Parkinson Disease Association
800-433-7022 National Parkinson Foundation
800-344-7872 Parkinson's Educational Program

Patients' Rights
617-769-5720 New England Patient's Rights Group, Inc.

Personal Hygiene
800-810-4000 Compliance Control Center

Porphyria
713-266-9617 American Porphyria Foundation

Premenstrual Syndrome
800-222-4767 PMS Access

Prenatal Care
800-673-8444 Healthy Mothers, Healthy Babies Coalition
800-433-5523 Be Healthy, Inc.

Prostatitis
309-664-6222 Prostatitis Foundation

Psoriasis
800-723-9166 National Psoriasis Foundation

Rare Diseases
203-746-6518 National Organization of Rare Disorders

Schizophrenia
800-847-3802 American Schizophrenia Association
516-829-0091 National Alliance for Research on
  Schizophrenia and Depression

Scleroderma
800-722-4673 United Scleroderma Foundation
800-441-CURE Scleroderma Research Foundation

Directory

Continued

Scoliosis

800-673-6922 National Scoliosis Foundation, Inc.

Sexually Transmitted Diseases

800-227-8922 National STD Hotline

Sickle Cell

800-421-8453 National Association for Sickle Cell Disease, Inc.

SIDS (Sudden Infant Death Syndrome)

800-221-SIDS National SIDS Alliance

Spina Bifida

800-621-3141 Spina Bifida Association

Spinal Cord Injuries

800-962-9629 National Spinal Cord Injury Association
800-526-3456 National Spinal Cord Injury Hotline

Stroke

800-553-6321 Courage Stroke Network
800-787-6537 National Stroke Association

Stuttering

800-221-2483 National Center for Stuttering

Thalassemia

800-522-7222 Thalassemia Action Group

Tourette Syndrome

800-237-0717 Tourette Syndrome Association

Wilson's Disease

800-399-0266 Wilson's Disease Association

Women's Health

310-410-9886 Findings: The Women's Health Care Advocacy Service

Directory

From: Miller/Keane: Encyclopedia & Dictionary of Medicine, Nursing, & Allied Health (6th ed.). Philadelphia: WB Saunders, p.1884-1886. Reprinted with permission.

Certified Poison Control Centers

ALABAMA

Alabama Poison Center, Tuscaloosa

408-A Paul Bryant Drive
Tuscaloosa, AL 35401
Emergency Phone:
(800) 462-0800 (AL only) or
(205) 345-0600

Regional Poison Control Center

The Children's Hospital of
Alabama
1600 Seventh Ave.
South Birmingham, AL 35233
Emergency Phone:
(205) 939-9201,
(800) 292-6678 (AL only) or
(205) 933-4050

ARIZONA

Arizona Poison and Drug Information Center

Arizona Health Sciences Center
Room #3204-K
1501 N. Campbell Ave.
Tucson, AZ 85724
Emergency Phone:
(800) 362-0101 (AZ only)
(602) 626-6016

Samaritan Regional Poison Center

Good Samaritan Regional Medical
Center, Ancillary-1
1111 E. McDowell Road
Phoenix, AZ 85006
Emergency Phone:
(602) 253-3334

CALIFORNIA

Central California Regional Poison Control Center

Valley Children's Hospital
3141 N. Millbrook, IN31
Fresno, CA 93703
Emergency Phone:
(800) 346-5922 (Central CA only)
(209) 445-1222

San Diego Regional Poison Center

UCSD Medical Center
200 West Arbor Drive
San Diego, CA 92103-8925
Emergency Phone:
(619) 543-6000,
(800) 876-4766 (619 area code only)

San Francisco Bay Area Regional Poison Control Center

San Francisco General Hospital
1001 Potrero Ave., Building 80,
Room 230
San Francisco, CA 94110
Emergency Phone:
(800) 523-2222

Santa Clara Valley Regional Poison Center

Valley Health Center, Suite 310
750 South Bascom Ave.
San Jose, CA 95128
Emergency Phone:
(408) 885-6000
(800) 662-9886 (CA only)

University of California, Davis Medical Center Regional Poison Control Center

2315 Stockton Blvd.
Sacramento, CA 95817
Emergency Phone:
(916) 734-3692;
(800) 342-9293 (Northern CA)

Continued

Directory

COLORADO

Rocky Mountain Poison and Drug Center

645 Bannock St.
Denver, CO 80204
Emergency Phone:
(303) 629-1123

DISTRICT OF COLUMBIA

National Capital Poison Center

3201 New Mexico Ave, NW
Suite 310
Washington, DC 20016
Emergency Numbers:
(202) 625-3333,
(202) 362-8563 (TTY)

FLORIDA

Florida Poison Information Center Jacksonville

655 West 8th Street
Jacksonville, FL 32209
Emergency Phone:
(904) 549-4480
(800) 282-3171 (FL only)

The Florida Poison Information and Toxicology Resource Center

Tampa General Hospital
Post Office Box 1289
Tampa, FL 33601
Emergency Phone:
(813) 253-4444 (Tampa)
(800) 282-3171 (Florida)

GEORGIA

Georgia Poison Center

Grady Memorial Hospital
80 Butler Street S.E.
P.O. Box 26066
Atlanta, GA 30335-3801
Emergency Phone:
(800) 282-5846 (GA only),
(404) 616-9000

INDIANA

Indiana Poison Center

Methodist Hospital of Indiana
1701 N. Senate Boulevard
P.O. Box 1367
Indianapolis, IN 46206-1367
Emergency Phone:
(800) 382-9097 (IN only),
(317) 929-2323

KENTUCKY

Kentucky Regional Poison Center of Kosair s Children s Hospital

P.O. Box 35070
Louisville, KY 40232-5070
Emergency Phone:
(502) 629-7275
(800) 722-5725 (KY only)

MARYLAND

Maryland Poison Center

20 N. Pine St.
Baltimore, MD 21201
Emergency Phone:
(410) 528-7701
(800) 492-2414 (MD only)

National Capital Poison Center (D.C. suburbs only)

3201 New Mexico Ave, NW
Suite 310
Washington, DC 20016
Emergency Numbers:
(202) 625-3333,
(202) 362-8563 (TTY)

MASSACHUSETTS

Massachusetts Poison Control System

300 Longwood Ave.
Boston, MA 02115
Emergency Phone:
(617) 232-2120,
(800) 682-9211

Continued

Directory

MICHIGAN
Poison Control Center
Children's Hospital of Michigan
3901 Beaubien Blvd.
Detroit, MI 48201
Emergency Phone:
(313) 745-5711

MINNESOTA
Hennepin Regional Poison Center
Hennepin County Medical Center
701 Park Ave.
Minneapolis, MN 55415
Emergency Phone:
(612) 347-3141,
Petline: (612) 337-7387,
TDD (612) 337-7474

Minnesota Regional Poison Center
St. Paul-Ramsey Medical Center
640 Jackson St.
St. Paul, MN 55101
Emergency Phone:
(612) 221-2113

MISSOURI
Cardinal Glennon Children s Hospital
Regional Poison Center
1465 S. Grand Blvd.
St. Louis, MO 63104
Emergency Phone:
(314) 772-5200,
(800) 366-8888

MONTANA
Rocky Mountain Poison and Drug Center
645 Bannock St.
Denver, CO 80204
Emergency Phone:
(303) 629-1123

NEBRASKA
The Poison Center
8301 Dodge St.
Omaha, NE 68114
Emergency Phone:
(402) 390-5555 (Omaha),
(800) 955-9119 (NE & WY)

NEW JERSEY
New Jersey Poison Information and Education System
201 Lyons Ave.
Newark, NJ 07112
Emergency Phone:
(800) 962-1253

NEW MEXICO
New Mexico Poison and Drug Information Center
University of New Mexico
Albuquerque, NM 87131-1076
Emergency Phone:
(505) 843-2551,
(800) 432-6866 (NM only)

NEW YORK
Hudson Valley Regional Poison Center
Phelps Memorial Hospital Center
701 North Broadway
North Tarrytown, NY 10591
Emergency Phone:
(800) 336-6997,
(914) 366-3030

Long Island Regional Poison Control Center
Winthrop University Hospital
259 First Street
Mineola, NY 11501
Emergency Phone:
(516) 542-2323, 542-2324,
542-2325, 542-3813

Directory

Continued

New York City Poison Control Center

N.Y.C. Department of Health
455 First Ave., Room 123
New York, NY 10016
Emergency Phone:
(212) 340-4494,
(212) P-O-I-S-O-N-S,
TDD (212) 689-9014

NORTH CAROLINA

Carolinas Poison Center

1000 Blythe Blvd.
P.O. Box 32861
Charlotte, NC 28232-2861
Emergency Phone:
(704) 355-4000
(800) 84-TOXIN,
(800-848-6946)

OHIO

Central Ohio Poison Center

700 Children's Drive
Columbus, OH 43205-2696
Emergency Phone:
(614) 228-1323
(800) 682-7625,
(614) 228-2272 (TTY),
(614) 461 -2012

Cincinnati Drug & Poison Information Center and Regional Poison Control System

231 Bethesda Avenue, M.L.
144 Cincinnati, OH 45267-0144
Emergency Phone:
(513) 558-5111,
(800) 872-5111 (OH only)

OREGON

Oregon Poison Center

Oregon Health Sciences University
3181 S.W. Sam Jackson Park Road
Portland, OR 97201
Emergency Phone:
(503) 494-8968,
(800) 452-7165 (OR only)

PENNSYLVANIA

Central Pennsylvania Poison Center

University Hospital
Milton S. Hershey Medical Center
Hershey, PA 17033
Emergency Phone:
(800) 521 -6110

The Poison Control Center serving the Greater Philadelphia metropolitan area

One Children's Center
Philadelphia, PA 19104-4303
Emergency Phone:
(215) 386-2100

Pittsburgh Poison Center

3705 Fifth Avenue
Pittsburgh, PA 15213
Emergency Phone:
(412) 681-6669

RHODE ISLAND

Rhode Island Poison Center

593 Eddy St.
Providence, Rl 02903
Emergency Phone:
(401) 277-5727

TEXAS

North Texas Poison Center

5201 Harry Hines Blvd.
P.O. Box 35926
Dallas, TX 75235
Emergency Phone:
(214) 590-5000,
Texas Watts (800) 441-0040

Directory

Continued

Southeast Texas Poison Center

The University of Texas Medical Branch
Galveston, TX 77550-2780
Emergency Phone:
(409) 765-1420 (Galveston),
(713) 654-1701 (Houston)

UTAH
Utah Poison Control Center

410 Chipeta Way, Suite 230
Salt Lake City, UT 84108
Emergency Phone:
(801) 581-2151,
(800) 456-7707 (UT only)

VIRGINIA
Blue Ridge Poison Center

Box 67 Blue Ridge Hospital
Charlottesville, VA 22901
Emergency Phone:
(804) 924-5543,
(800) 451-1428

National Capital Poison Center (Northern VA only)

3201 New Mexico Ave, NW
Suite 310
Washington, DC 20016
Emergency Numbers:
(202) 625-3333,
(202) 362-8563 (TTY)

WEST VIRGINIA
West Virginia Poison Center

3110 MacCorkle Ave. S.E.
Charleston, WV 25304
Emergency Phone:
(800) 642-3625 (WV only)
(304) 348-4211

WYOMING
The Poison Center

8301 Dodge St.
Omaha, NE 68114
Emergency Phone:
(402) 390-5555 (Omaha),
(800) 955-9119 (NE & WY)

From: Miller/Keane: Encyclopedia & Dictionary of Medicine, Nursing, & Allied Health (6th ed.). Philadelphia: WB Saunders, p.1887-1888. Reprinted with permission.

Directory

USEFUL INTERNET ADDRESSES

Description	Web Address	Notes

INTERESTING BOOKS/JOURNALS

Description	Title/Author	Publisher/Year

NOTES

Directory

A
B

C
D

C
D

E
F

G
H

G
H

I
J

I
J

K
L

K
L

M
N

M
N

O
P

O
P

Q
R

Q
R

S
T

**S
T**

S
T

S
T

U
V

U
V

W
X

Thurs Aug 15th

11:00

Susan Irvine

Howsov

Y
Z

Excelior

Camp Based

excelsior (Health and

Safety Computer Based

exams CD.

101

Saunders Camp Review

RN-NClex.